GRATEFUL GUILT

LIVING IN THE SHADOW OF MY HEART

STEVEN G. TAIBBI

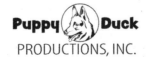
Puppy Duck
PRODUCTIONS, INC.

This book is dedicated to my two heart donors, Lawrence (I never learned his last name) and David Jocobo and their families who made the donations possible. You all have my eternal gratitude.

It is also dedicated to all donors of every type and their families who have enough love, in the face of personal tragedy, to see through their pain and help others. What could be greater than that?

*Without donors and donation,
transplantation is just a wish.
God speed.*

CONTENTS

INTRODUCTION

Sometimes life isn't easy. This book is about a life full of physical, emotional and spiritual challenges. It is the story of my husband, Steven, a man I adore and admire, a man who has learned to accept his challenges and confront them; a man with incredible strength.

For years I thought his story should be told. Some of the memories were difficult for him, but his goal in writing this book is to share the strategies he used to deal with the cards life dealt him. Perhaps his strategies can be used by others to confront their own difficulties. When people are sick or struggling through tough times, they often receive suggestions on how to deal with their situation. The strategies in this book are from someone who has personal experience and has "walked the walk." For those who are not sick but are dealing with someone who is or experiencing their own struggles not necessarily related to health, this book will show you how to live life to the fullest and to keep a positive attitude and how to confront whatever it is you are confronting head-on.

Steven's troubles began as a young child and continue to this day. The book begins with a young child as he faces his first life and death situation. This is the true story of a boy growing up in a time when adults believed children would not understand and didn't need explanations. As a result, he was most often not given any information to help ease his fears of what was happening. Some of the stories told speak of individuals who made tough situations tougher instead of easier. They are not a reflection of how everyone would handle the situation; but these are stories of what happened to him. Steven decided very early on to take control and, amazingly, found ways to confront and deal with what life presented him. Children can be good teachers and there are lessons to be learned from these stories. I have learned so much from him – about life, about strength, about attitude and about what is really important.

I have always been amazed by his sense of humor. Even during the toughest moments he has made me laugh. He has a gift for making others feel better when he is the one doing the suffering. In addition to his sense of humor is his ability to be sympathetic and empathic about problems others are facing. He actually thinks his health struggles during our marriage have been tougher on me! Of course, I don't see it that way since I have witnessed much of what he has been through. His attitude made things much easier for me and his humor and ability to laugh made many situations easier for both of us. I have always believed that in the midst of tragedy come many blessings. My husband's story is no different. There have been many blessings– though sometimes we had to stop for a moment to find them.

I hope you enjoy Steven's book as much as I have. It's a good read. I also hope that you gain from it lessons you might need.

God Bless.

Rose M. Taibbi

1

They've been cutting into me since the day I was born—and they still haven't stopped. Unlike most people who have had a heart transplant, or heart attack for that matter, their need for a transplant—or the event of a heart attack—was often the first time they have ever needed major surgery. Many recipients, not just of hearts, but of other organs as well, have told me that the failure of an organ was the first time they had ever been seriously ill.

Not me. When I was born on April 26, 1953, I was *cyanotic*, doctor-speak for what was commonly called a "blue baby." That means that at birth my heart wasn't pumping efficiently enough to properly oxygenate my blood, hence the bluish hue I greeted the world with.

I was also born with two birth defects that required three operations to correct. The first, and most embarrassing, but also the one to have the least effect on my life, was that I was born with a closed penis. A couple of snips later and I was good as new.

The other birth defects were more serious; on both of my hands the thumbs were crooked. They bent at the first knuckle towards the left. If I put my hands together, one thumb next to the other, they fit into each other perfectly, like two lovers spooning. I can bend my left thumb at the first knuckle most of the way; the right thumb is fixed at the first joint. The doctors were concerned that a tendon was pulling them out of place; as a result, they cut along the entire length outside of each thumb and cut the suspected tendons. It wouldn't be until forty-six years later that I would learn the real reason why I was born with these three defects and what they had to do with the, as of yet, undiscovered defects in my heart.

At the time, all this meant to my parents, and later to me when I was old enough to understand such things, was that April 26th was not only the anniversary of my birth, but also the anniversary of my first three operations. It was also the beginning of a life-long guilt-trip for my mother, who, till the day she died, never stopped blaming herself for the condition of the only child she would ever give birth to.

2

My parents took me to their home in Malverne, Long Island to live with them and my two older adopted brothers, Peter and Michael. Then, a couple of years later, my parents also adopted my younger sister, Neiani. All three of my siblings were what were called "troubled adoptions." Peter was over four years of age and had been bounced around from one foster home to another when Salvatore and Gaetana Taibbi finally brought him to a home he could call his own. Michael was three. His birth mother was white and his father Pilipino. My sister was almost two when she had been brought into the family, and she was half Chinese and half European. You have to give my parents credit—this was the fifties, after all. Two non-white children was a big deal back then.

It didn't take long for my mother's guilt to dramatically change the dynamics of the family. Mom was a nurse, and her nursing instincts kicked in immediately in all matters concerning my health. She started to put up a protective "fence" around herself and me, and as time grew so did the fence. In a few years to come, it would grow high enough that no other member of the family would be able jump it. Including me. The family had started to become one that consisted of two camps—Mom and me in one, the rest of the family in the other. The seeds of the understandable resentment this caused in both my siblings and my father began to take root, along with the seeds of guilt that started to grow in me as I began to blame myself for the family situation.

To say that I was an underweight child would be an understatement. I was alarmingly thin, and my mother heard that alarm with astute clarity. My mother knew deep in her nurse's bones that physically there was something seriously wrong with me. To my mother's eternal frustration, doctors didn't seem to agree, and she took all matters concerning my health into her own hands. Mom went into battle mode, convinced that I was in grave danger and the doctors be damned. My survival became her main concern and she was going to do everything in her power to keep me alive long enough until such time that a doctor, any doctor, somewhere, sometime, would be able to see the same danger stalking me that she did. By the time I was four my mother was making her own concoctions of "health drinks" for me to consume. The only two ingredients of this drink I can remember now were milk and raw eggs, but I remember there were others. I recall that the whitish-yellow mixture that came out of the blender tasted good and that I enjoyed these drinks and had one every morning "to keep my strength up," as my mother would say.

Mom also noticed that I seemed to crave sugar and her nursing instincts told her that my body was telling us both something. Consequently, I had an endless supply of hard candy to suck on as often as I wanted. To my mother, this craving was another way my body was asking for something "to keep my strength up."

As it turns out, where matters of my health were concerned, Mom was right about all of it.

3

When I was five, there was a suspicion that my grandfather, who was living with us, might have tuberculosis. As a precaution, doctors suggested that the whole family needed to have X-rays taken. All I remember of the day when I had my X-ray was that it was mild outside and that the building I walked into while holding my mother's hand had black glass doors with some white block writing on them. I remember being happy and enjoying the nice weather. A few days later my parents were given the results by Dr. Camardella, a wonderful gentleman who had a family practice a block and a half directly up the street from our suburban home.

I wasn't there when my parents were given the news; at least I don't think I was, but from that moment on, nothing would ever be the same again, as the life I had known quickly dissolved in an acid-bath of panic and frantic action. Suddenly, my existence no longer revolved around my home, toys, and the life and family I always knew as my world. Instead, it had been replaced by a flurry of doctors and tests, and the confusion and shame of complete strangers removing my clothes while armed with needles, blood pressure cuffs and stethoscopes.

In those days, children were treated very differently than they are today and that includes even those who were patients. Back then, sick children were invisible as actual people to both parents and doctors. This was the 50's, 1958 to be exact, and children were "to be seen and not heard." Doctors, nurses and techs would come into an exam or hospital room, strangers, people I had never seen before, and just remove my clothing, conduct tests or exams and, most times, never introduce themselves, never ask permission and never explain what they were about to do to me. If they spoke, it was with as few words as possible; just enough to get me to do what they wanted. My dignity was not a concern. Why would it be? After all, I was just a kid. What did I know? It didn't end there. While I didn't have the sophistication to express it then, I certainly felt, and understood, that in a bizarre and almost supernatural way my illness had taken away my person-hood and transformed me into a piece of meat that had a problem that needed to be solved. More oddly still, I had become a piece of meat without ears. Doctors and my parents would talk about my situation right in front of me as if I wasn't even there, assured somehow that I didn't comprehend what was being said because I didn't yet have a good enough grasp of the language to understand what they were saying. Often, during these exams, and later in the hospital, I would imagine I was a giant log of salami. They were only partially correct in their assumptions. I may not have known what all the "big words" meant, but I sure got the gist. Body language, tone and facial expressions are a universal language, known even by small children. I easily gleaned enough to I know I was in trouble, big trouble, but because no one thought I had any idea of what was going on, no one did anything to assuage my fears or perceptions. How wrong they were. No one, *no one*, told me anything.

Through all this, my now-vindicated mother became even more earnest in her battle to fight for my survival. Her face took on a new expression: sterner, more purposeful and deeply skeptical. The doctors had been wrong, she had been right. From here on in, there was a new sheriff in town, and any more misdiagnosis or treatments were not to be tolerated. She wore this expression as a warning, and all medical personnel had better take heed. Those who didn't, did at their own peril. Ironically, this attitude didn't always serve me well.

What had set all this in motion, of course, was what they found on the X-rays. Dr. Camardella told my parents that fortunately, while no one in the family had tuberculosis, there was a problem, a serious problem, with my little five-year-old heart. The X-ray clearly showed a "grossly enlarged heart." When a heart is enlarged, it not only means that the heart is larger than it should be, but, more importantly, that the heart is no longer able to pump efficiently. What was causing this enlargement had yet to be determined. Doctor Camardella referred us to the best pediatric cardiologist he knew of, Edgar P. Mannix, Jr., who had recently moved from Houston, Texas, to Long Island.

Turns out, not only had Mom been right all along that there was something seriously wrong with me, but now her worst fears, the unspeakable, was confirmed as well. In my first visit to his Garden City, New York office, my parents were told there was no time to spare. According to Dr Mannix, I was near death and the cause of the enlargement had to be ascertained immediately, and, if possible, corrected immediately after that. I can only imagine how shocking this must have been to my parents. I can only imagine all the "I told you so's" my father had to endure from my mother. In any case, it had to be nothing short of a bomb going off in the middle of their lives.

For me, the suddenness of the situation was stunning, almost incomprehensible. In what seemed to be in the blink of an eye, I was whisked away from the comfort of my home and everything and everyone I knew, and on June 9th, 1958, at 10:10 in the morning, I was brought to and deposited into the confines of St. Francis Hospital in Roslyn, New York. I don't remember the admitting process, or how I found myself in my first hospital gown, or where my clothes went. All I knew was I went in there as a five-year-old kid who had a family and toys and my own clothes back home, as well as the ones that had recently been on my back, but then suddenly found myself in a ward of twelve identical beds, including mine, with nothing, not anything at all, of my own. I had been stripped of everything.

Each bed was occupied with other children who also had heart problems—all of us being tended by nuns, (most of whom were nurses) lay nurses and doctors—in that order. I was now a stranger in a new, completely alien world, filled with sights and sounds I had never experienced before.

The hospital was frightening and cold by its nature, if not by actual temperature, and, in the worst sense of the word, the very definition of "institutional." The room was huge, stark, and had giant white block walls and high ceilings with sheer white curtains on the large windows that did nothing to soften the severity of the room. There were no decorations of any kind save for a very large crucifix and an autoclave, if either can be classified as "decorations." The bed frames were made of square tubing that was coated in white ceramic–just like that found on ceramic kitchen sinks. Because of our age, the side rails were up, and for all intents and purposes, it felt like a prison. Based on the time of my admission, I know I had to have had at least two meals there that day, but I don't remember them. Also, I'm sure that I must've gone to the bathroom at least a couple of times, too, but I don't remember that, either. I do know that we weren't allowed out of bed, so it was also the day I was introduced to the bedpan.

The whole experience was not only emotionally crushing, worse, it had ripped any dignity I might have had away from my small, five-year-old personhood. Being half naked, having to use bedpans in front of complete strangers, having no single object that was mine, all of this, combined with the fear, the newness and strangeness of it all, somehow mixed together and produced a new and deeply disturbing emotion: shame. It might have been new then, and I would never get used to it, but from that day all the way until now, shame would dog me, follow me, find me and keep me company even when I wanted to be alone.

The one thing I remember most vividly, however, was my mother's parting instruction to me before she and my father left. Tomorrow, I was told, I was going to have my first procedure, although I'm sure that wasn't the way she put it. I wouldn't have breakfast because they were going to use something called anesthesia, and that this anesthesia was going to make me go to sleep. They were going to give it to me through a mask, just like Buck Rogers wore in his space ship. I liked Buck Rogers, didn't I? Yes. So, if I had breakfast and they put this mask on me and I had eaten breakfast that morning, the anesthesia would make me throw-up in my mask while I was sleeping, and I could choke to death– *on my own vomit*. Now we don't want that to happen, do we? NO. But most of all, she told me in my final instructions, I was to be a good boy. I was to listen to the doctors and nurses and not complain and always behave. I was to do whatever I was told and not fight or resist. I was to be a good boy. I was to be–*a good boy*. I didn't have to worry, everything would be fine, and they would be there when I woke up. After my parting instructions, hugs and kisses, heartfelt expressions that they loved me, and further promises that they would be back the next day, my parents departed and left me alone to my new reality.

I had never slept in a room that large before, or one that, even with the lights off, was that bright. Strange sounds, some human, others not, along with the smell of disinfectant and frightened children, intertwined and permeated the air and populated it like some living and yet un-seeable thing whose tentacles surrounded me and my bed, lacing through the bedrails, which offered no protection, hissing menacingly in my ears as they brushed over my face.

The bedrails. What an effect those bedrails had. I'm fairly sure my hospital bed was about the same size as my bed at home, but this bed felt enormous, and no matter which direction I looked from my pillow, I was looking through rails—make that bars. White prison bars. I never felt so small.

If my bed and the walls, floors and ceiling had been made of stone, like those dungeons I had seen in my Sir Lancelot comic books, it couldn't have felt any colder, more foreign or more terrifying.

Frightened and feeling more alone than at any other time in my young life, I lay down on my side and curled-up into the fetal position and rocked myself to sleep—something I still do to this day. It was that night when I found the entrance to my cave.

4

I woke to the sounds of breakfast being served to the ward. Nuns and orderlies were busy taking trays out of stainless steel carts, lowering bed railings to a height that would allow the over-bed tables to be maneuvered and swung into place, and placing trays on the tables. Most of the sounds were metallic in nature, the bed railings, the tray tables, the carts and clinking silverware. These sounds were accompanied by the smell of the food, and while the sounds had awakened me, the smell of the food brought into sharp focus how hungry I was.

I looked at the bed across from mine. He wasn't being served food either, and that's when I saw it: a sign hanging from the top of his footboard that read, NO FOOD. The two words were stacked vertically, big, bright red letters with white boarders on a black background, in a stainless-steel frame. I looked to my footboard, and I could see the back of a stainless-steel frame through the bars of my bed. I got out from under the covers and went to it. The frame had a wide, flat hook on it that exactly fit the square tubing of my bed. I un-hooked it and took it into my hands, saw that it had the same message as the one across from me, turned it over and over, examined it for a short while and, being a good boy, put it back, exactly in the center of the foot-board where I had found it.

They came for my neighbor first. Two men, orderlies, dressed in white from head to foot, came through the large double doors that were opposite me, guiding a gurney with them. I thought they looked like milkmen. They lowered the rails and brought the gurney to the side of the bed, whose occupant started to cry and protest. I turned away. I no longer wanted to watch. As his cries dimmed as they went through the doors, I thought to myself, I won't cry. I won't protest. I'm a good boy.

They came for me a little while later. They lowered the rails, brought the gurney alongside and slid me onto it. Then they did something I didn't expect. Had I watched them take my neighbor it wouldn't have been such a surprise, but I had averted my eyes too soon to see this next step. They tied me down. My arms were put into little wrist-cuffs made of leather and lined with what had to be lamb's wool with a double buckle to cinch it closed. They then did the same to my ankles. I wondered about this because I was being a good boy. I hadn't made a sound. I hadn't struggled in the least. I don't remember them saying anything to me. They might have, but nothing that left any impression. They were just there to collect me. It wasn't explained to me that this was for my own safety.

I was delivered to the operating room. By this time, I'd barely been in the hospital 24 hours. The difference between my being home just a day ago and what I now found to be my current circumstance were absolutely incomprehensible to me. I was unstrapped from the gurney and slid over onto the operating table. I can't recollect ten words being spoken during this whole process. I never said a single word. Not one. Once again, my arms and legs were strapped down, this time under the enormous operating room light that was directly above me.

There was a soft buzz of conversation in the room, muffled by the face masks everyone was wearing. There was a quiet tinkling sound being made as the surgical instruments were being prepared. Everyone was wearing long, white, surgical gowns that matched their face masks. The gowns and masks were made of cloth. The odor of disinfectant was strong, but it was accompanied by a more subtle smell, and it wasn't pleasant. It made my empty stomach turn a little. In a few minutes I would find out just what that smell was.

Then a man wearing a mask with a matching surgical cap bent down over me. He started to speak to me, and his voice was soft and gentle. He was going to put the mask on me, like the one Buck Rogers wore, so I knew that this man and my parents had spoken. As the mask came towards my face, it filled my entire vision. It looked enormous. I can still see that mask coming at me today. He put the mask on my face and told me to count to ten and to breathe normally. God, the smell! Ether! It made me want to gag, to cough. The smell was horrible, and along with it, I could smell the rubber the mask was made of, which was an unpleasant enough smell on its own. It made me want to rip the mask off, but I didn't even try. And that wasn't because I was tied down. At this point I'd forgotten that. No, that wasn't it; that didn't matter.

I lay perfectly still because I was a good boy. So, I did what I was told to do: I counted. One. Two. Three. Four. My head was beginning to spin. Five. Six. The smell was making me nauseous; I felt panic swelling in me, and I thought, *I'm going to get sick in my mask! I'm going to choke! I'll die on my own vomit and I didn't even eat breakfast!* Seven. Eight. The room started to blur and spin even more. Then everything started to go dark. Nin.... I didn't count any higher.

5

The headache. Oh, my God, the headache. I'd never had such a powerful headache before in my entire life. And the nausea. It equaled the headache in its intensity and everything was still spinning, sickeningly spinning.

That's what it was like coming out of anesthesia in the late fifties. You simply felt awful and that was that. I woke up with sandbags on my groin to keep pressure on the wounds. (Don't you just love it that doctor-speak for an incision they've given you is a "wound?" Personally, I think it's a hoot.) They hurt. I'm fairly sure I woke up back in my ward, but I was so disoriented that I could be wrong about that. I'm also fairly sure I woke up alone. I don't recall my parents being there. Back then, visitors came at visiting time only. I could be wrong, but I don't remember them being there when I finally came to. I'm sure somebody was there to tell me I wouldn't be allowed to move for fear of tearing the stitches that had closed my femoral artery. I would have to lay there flat without moving for hours. And, for all I knew, I was still tied down.

But the cardiac catheterization had gone well, in the sense that I had tolerated the procedure well enough and they had discovered the cause of my enlarged heart. Again, I wasn't there when the doctors told my parents what they had discovered, but the news was dire. I can't imagine what this would have done to Mom and Dad, but I'm sure of one thing: It had to be a powerful blow to them both.

Cardiac catheterizations are a routine procedure today. Usually done under a local anesthetic and sometimes a mild sedative, you are awake for the procedure and you go home the same day. It was a much bigger deal back then, as the fact that they used to put you under underscores. But the basic idea is the same. After they put me out, a four-inch cut was made in either my right or left groin to gain entry to the femoral artery. Once they had access, a catheter was inserted and fed up the artery to both the right and left side of the heart. The procedure is done under a fluoroscope, a type of X-ray that doesn't just take a snapshot picture like the X-ray your doctor holds up to the light, but instead, shows a live image of what it's focused on for as long as the machine is running. They used this to help guide the catheters from my groin all the way up into the heart, and then used it to look at the heart itself. If this was a modern procedure, they would also inject a dye at this time with a radioactive signature that can be seen on the fluoroscope, which in turn allows them to see, in real time, the functioning of the heart. That part of the procedure is called an angiogram. But, this was back then. I had to have two procedures while today the whole thing can be done with one in as little as 20 minutes. The catheterization was being done to measure the pressures in each chamber of the heart and to measure the amount of oxygen in the interior cardiac blood, and more than likely, to take an interior blood sample. The results of my catheterization had relayed the worst news possible.

I had been born, my parents were told, with a deformed heart. I had two atrial septum defects, or ASD's. The common name for my condition back then was "a hole in the heart." What that meant was that at the time of my birth, my heart had yet to finish forming. The wall between the upper chambers of the heart, the left and right atriums, hadn't fully closed and there was leakage between them. It was found that one of the ASD's was "with a huge left to right shunt." This was causing the pumping action of the heart to be extremely inefficient, would only get worse, and in *the very near future*, certainly cause my death. But wait! There's more, as they say in TV land. I also had something called "partial anomalous pulmonary venous drainage." Doctor speak for one of the major veins was plumbed backwards, entering at the wrong place in my heart. This was also very bad news, as one could easily imagine.

I see in my mind's eye my parents being completely dumbfounded at this news. They were being told that their only natural born child was at death's door and the prognosis was poor at best. I'm sure even though the fact that I was deathly ill was what my mother had been fearing all along, the confirmation of her worst fears must have knocked the legs right out from under her. That really had to be something for my poor parents to digest, don't you think? I wonder what they told my brothers and sister. I wonder what it was like when they were finally alone at home that night. I wonder if they went into my bedroom and just stood there looking at my empty bed. I wonder what it was like back home. I still wonder.

Two days later, an almost identical scenario was played out. Now they were going to perform the angiogram where they insert a catheter and this time, inject the dye. I woke to a bed that had the NO FOOD placard on the footboard again, just as it was only two days ago. I didn't get to eat breakfast that day either. They came to get me and wheeled me into an operating room and once again strapped me to the table. Once again, they would put me out with a gas mixture that contained the now dreaded ether.

Now to be honest, I can't be certain if during the first procedure they cut me only once in one groin, and now I was going to get the second cut, or if they were going to go back into what were two existing cuts. If I had to bet on it, I think during this second procedure I would receive the second cut. Either way, I ended that day with two four-inch incisions, one on each side of my groin.

If I had found the entrance to my cave my first night in the hospital, three days later, I had climbed into it. I was a hurting little boy, both emotionally and physically. Sure, by the time I had been admitted to St. Francis, I'd been operated on three times, but those operations had been performed on the day I was born. I didn't remember anything about them. But I sure remembered the NO FOOD sign and what it meant two days ago—not being fed breakfast, being strapped to gurneys and operating tables, the ether. I remembered how I felt coming out of anesthesia, sandbags atop my groin, not being able to move. I remembered being in pain. I remember waking up and how my body had been changed. I hadn't known that was going to happen. I was told I'd be like Buck Rogers, wearing his mask during a space mission. It's like I said earlier, they really weren't that good with children. But most of all, I remembered my parents' instructions: Be a good boy. Don't fight, don't complain, don't resist. *Be a good boy.* How was I to do what my parents wanted when all of this was awful? And I wanted very badly not to let them down. I didn't want to disappoint my mother, and I wanted to be a man for my father. What could I do to not complain when there was much to rationally complain about? What was I to do?

My cave was the answer. My cave. Coming out of the anesthesia, hurting and not being allowed to move had started the earnest, mental digging of my cave. I think psychologists would have called it disassociation. I called it survival.

I had carved this cave in my mind. I can still see it clearly today, still see me in it as I was then. When I visualized me in my cave, I would see it as if I was outside of myself and could see me in it, as if the part seeing me in my cave was just some disinterested individual looking at something of no particular interest. I saw myself from the side, a cut-away view, as you do when looking at an ant farm. For me to be in that cave, I needed the disinterested me looking in. The disinterested me, who couldn't feel anything, also somehow protected the part of me in the cave from feeling anything. The guardian me. After a while, I didn't have to see from the disinterested me point of view, but I knew that he was always there.

So, by a combination of accident and necessity, I had come up with my first strategy: a little frightened boy's first tactic to cope with the pain, the terror and the *loneliness* of my situation. I haven't used the cave in decades, but to this day I try to disassociate myself from whatever new situation my health puts me in. Nowadays, I usually put myself in my friend's sloop, under sail on a beautiful, windy day on Long Island Sound. I hear the wind, the flapping of the sail, the seagulls and the rushing of the water as the boat slices through it. I feel the warmth of the sun on my face and the motion of the vessel. It's not quite as effective as my cave was, but it's a mentally healthier way to make procedures more bearable.

The cave I had expertly visualized for myself had a slope

along the front that contained the entrance. It was made entirely of solid, dark grey rock. It looked wet, but it wasn't. It looked cold, but it was warm and snug. I would crawl in, and later, as I got better at it, I was able to just find myself in it, sitting with my legs drawn up, my arms tight around my legs, rocking, just rocking, like I did that first night to go to sleep—like I still do. The small space that I occupied in my cave could just barely fit me, as if the cave, too, was holding me, and the top of the space I was in was below the entrance, even if someone looked in, they wouldn't or couldn't see me. Here, I was safe. Here, they couldn't hurt me, and I could feel no pain. Staying in my cave made it so I wouldn't fight, complain or resist. Here, in my cave, in complete disassociation of what was happening to me, the physical me was allowed to be a good boy. This almost worked too well, as further down the road, it nearly cost me my life.

So, this time, when they had come to get me, all they got was my body. I had the same reaction to the anesthesia and all the rest of it as I'd had two days ago. But this time I wasn't there, only my body was, and without me being in my body, me, *the actual me*, I didn't feel anything. I had found the way to please my parents, survive and most of all, be a good boy.

The angiogram only confirmed what they already knew, but now they could see the problem better and find a way to get in there and attempt a repair. It was bad. I was close to the edge, and my only chance was open-heart surgery for ASD repair. The game was on.

6

June 17, 1958 was the big day, exactly seven days from admission, and the doctors were going to "crack me open" in what was the vernacular then, as it is now, for open-heart surgery. But a lot had happened in the five days since my last procedure. At that time, the survival rate for ASD repair was around 50 percent. And that was just for a single ASD repair without a pulmonary venous malformation to further complicate things. This whole area was cutting-edge stuff. During the time I spent in that ward, a total of one month exactly, not counting time I spent in recovery and critical care, I saw children who would leave for surgery and never come back. For some reason, and I'm eternally grateful for this, my mother never lied to me about what had happened to those who never came back. They didn't come back because they were never coming back. Ever.

There was a terrifying incident with the boy whose bed was directly opposite mine, the one on whose footboard I first saw the placard NO FOOD. One day, in the time before my last procedure and my first open heart, I woke to see NO FOOD hanging from his bed. I quickly checked my footboard and was greatly relieved to find there was no placard there. While I ate breakfast the men who looked like milkmen came for him. He wanted no part of it. He had dark hair, looked to be in better condition than me, and was about the same height. They pulled the gurney up next to his bed, lowered the railing and he saw his chance. Like a shot, he had jumped out of bed between the small space between the gurney and the bed and made a run for it. The orderly at the head of the gurney wasn't quite fast enough to catch him, and as his arm swung to try to cut him off, he missed and all he caught was the wake this kid left behind him. But the orderly's futile attempt to catch him forced him to change direction, and he had nowhere to go but to the other side of the bed. The other orderly made a move to box him in between his bed and his neighbor's, but he ducked and got past. By this time the first orderly had positioned himself at the foot of the bed and just scooped him up not two steps later. The orderly held him to his chest, arms crossed over the boy whose feet and arms flailed as he continued screaming in protest. By this time every eye in that ward was glued to the surreal commotion playing out in front of us. I was frozen in horror while my mind raced at a million miles an hour. They finally got him on the gurney, strapped him down and started to leave. The large double doors next to his bed closed, but I could still hear the screams coming from way down the hall.

That was probably the first time I had ever been shaken down to my very core. I thought about him all day. When my parents finally came during visiting hours, I told them about the incident. It was apparent by my mother's body language that she already knew. Head down, her voice both soft and sad, my mother told me that he didn't make it. As she told me, I could hear her subtext: Her fear for my life was looming in front of all of us. I can still see that scene today. I can still see him. I still think about him. I wish I knew his name.

A few days later, I woke to see the sign on my bed. I knew it would be there because my parents had told me I'd have to be like Buck Rogers again but seeing it there this time terrified me. All I could think about was that little boy from a few days ago. I didn't want to go either. I hatched a plan. I knew that if I had breakfast they wouldn't be able to take me. So, I quietly got out from under my covers, slinked over to the footboard and took the sign. I put it close to my chest so others couldn't see that I had it, and, as surreptitiously as I could, got back under the covers and hid the sign under the blankets with me.

But I didn't feel safe. I was worried about the big weak spot in my plan. What if I had breakfast and they came and took me anyway? What if because I'd had breakfast and they gave me anesthesia, I would throw up in my mask and choke to death on my own vomit? This image grew brighter and brighter in my mind until I couldn't stand it anymore. So, I did the most difficult thing I had ever done in my young life. Feeling like I had been beaten, ashamed at my own powerlessness, I got out of the covers, put the sign back where I found it, and as I crawled back under the covers, I crawled into my cave. But even my cave could not protect me from the fact that the act of putting back that sign had broken me; broken me in a way that would haunt me my whole life.

7

oming out of anesthesia is a lot like floating to the surface after nearly drowning. You "come to," eyelids as heavy as anvils, in a sickening fog of leftover anesthesia, dizzy and disoriented. Breathing is difficult, and your throat hurts. This was a much worse experience than when the anesthesia had been for simple procedures, now I had been under for hours, five or six of them. My chest had been cut open from just below the center of the collar bone to a few inches above my navel. My sternum had been sawed in half vertically and a rib-spreader used to keep my chest open enough to have access to my heart. I had "cut downs," little one-to-two-inch incisions in the crooks of my elbows, at my wrists and ankles, as well as large ones in my groin, that I could have what was called back then, a pump-oxygenator, or a heart-lung machine as it's called today, hooked-up to me so that it could take blood from my body, add oxygen to it, and circulate the blood back to my body. This machine took over the functions of my heart and lungs so that the doctors could stop my heart while they made the repair. I was told the pump-oxygenator needed 24 pints of blood just to prime it. During the course of the operation, I used many more pints than that. My father, who was the national art director for AT&T, had written an appeal in the company newsletter asking co-workers for blood donations. Many of them stepped-up to the call and the blood bank received an excess of donations on my behalf. Thank you, AT&T. I will always have a soft spot in my heart for the company that AT&T was in those days.

I was in a great deal of pain, but between the leftover anesthesia and what had to be a massive dose of pain killers, it was if the pain were being "phoned-in" from a distance, which, while the pain was still powerful—dull and throbbing—at least I was not in agony. There was something else, too. I was inside an oxygen tent. Today, when you need oxygen, it's usually administered through a nasal cannula, a loop of plastic tubing that goes around your head, hooks over your ears and has two prongs that go into your nose. In the fifties, the medical technology solution for the problem of giving patients additional oxygen was a tent. Made of clear plastic, it was literally a rectangular tent that fit around the patient, down to about the middle thigh, and sat atop the bed and blankets. You can imagine how much oxygen must have escaped from such a contrivance, and because of that it made any kind of ignition source a genuine danger. Good thing I didn't smoke.

Clear plastic is really a misnomer; the plastic was similar to that used for automotive convertible rear windows. So, it was crinkly, which distorted your view, and like most convertible rear windows, it wasn't really clear as much as it was partially opaque. All this added to the confusion that is inherent when coming out of an anesthetic state.

One thing was familiar, however, and it was a lifeline that I desperately needed at that moment. My mother was sitting next to me, her hand under the tent, holding mine. My mother's familiar and soft hand felt like heaven; no, better yet, home. It reconnected me to a world that seemed to exist only in a distant memory. I remember seeing a distorted image of my father standing at the foot of my bed and some kind of exclamation between them at the event of my eyes opening. But it wouldn't last for long. I may have come back from being under. I may have come back from those unknown depths where someone under anesthesia goes and that science—even today can't explain, can't quantify, can't tell you where you go. It's not sleep, not a coma. The you that is you gets parked somewhere, and no one knows where that somewhere is or what you do while you're there. My eyes were heavy; I knew I had made it back from that unknown place. My parents were there, but all I wanted to do was escape from the pain. As I held my mother's hand, I drifted off into deep, merciful, and pain-free sleep.

8

The days that followed immediately after are lost to me. I just know I spent them in the Intensive Care Unit, or ICU. Today ICU's are known as the Critical Care Unit, or CCU. But what was true here was true of all the time I spent at St. Francis. You just lay there. There was no television, no music, no playing, not that I was in any mood or condition to play. You spent your day alone in bed. Think about how a five-year-old would experience lying in bed 24 hours a day with no source of entertainment or distraction. The time seemed interminable. Days seemed like weeks and weeks seemed like months. As a matter of fact, for most of my life, actually until I did research for this book and got my old records from the hospital, I thought that each of my stays at St. Francis were a year long, when in fact, the first stay was a month exactly and the second 30 days. But that is what it feels like and when you are five, a month is a much bigger chunk of your life than it is when you are in your sixties.

But even though I had tolerated the operation well enough—

a minor miracle in its own right—I wasn't doing as well as the doctors would have liked. What I didn't know was the operation had been only partially successful with the repair of only one of the holes. The other hole and the venous drainage problems still remained.

X-rays taken the next day seemed to show a fluid build-up in the right hemi thorax. I also had an electrocardiogram (what is commonly called an EKG) that day that didn't satisfy the doctors, either. EKG's show the electrical activity of the heart, which is gauged by the non-invasive use of electrodes attached to the skin, and then measured exactly in terms of how the heart is beating, its rhythm, and where weakness in the heart muscle may be located, if there is any.

Today, an EGK machine is literally the size of a laptop computer. You are connected to the machine through 12 wires, or *leads*, and they are attached by sticky, disposable pads fitted to the ends—the *electrodes*. You lay still for a few seconds as the tech operating the EKG pushes a button, and then you are done. The machine then prints out a graph, not unlike what you'd see in a polygraph test, for the doctor to study, record and compare against past and future EKG's. Modern hospitals have many of these machines.

This was not my first EKG. My first had been during that flurry of activity right after I had been diagnosed with an enlarged heart before I was admitted to the hospital. St. Francis had their EKG, yes, they only had one back then, in the basement. I can still see the rough, painted walls and the pipes hanging from the ceiling in the corridors of that basement. The machine was the size of a player piano, and the room that it was in was small, only large enough for the EKG and an examination bed. It had large round dials made of Bakelite and looked like something out of Frankenstein's own workshop. It was more fascinating than scary, however. It was a four-channel machine, a channel being where each lead terminated at the machine. Instead of pads for the electrodes, like those of today, the connections to your body were made by what for all the world looked like small brass bells, each about the size of a shot glass. They spread a conductive gel over the area they were going to measure, fixed the bells to a red rubber strap, placed the bells over the goop, and strapped that around you to hold it in place. As an aside, this red rubber was ubiquitous in medicine back then. I mean, it was *everywhere*. Certain kinds of tubing, enema bags, hot water bottles, all kinds of stuff, was made with this red rubber. When it did eventually get old, it would crack and ultimately fall apart. Whenever I think back to those days, that red rubber and glass syringes are invariably part of the memory.

It was not uncommon for a bell to slip during the test, forcing the tech conducting the test to stop what he was doing, reposition it, and then do that section of the test over again. While they were taking each measurement, you would have to lie perfectly still, and I mean *perfectly* still, until that portion of the test was over. Each measurement lasted at least 20 seconds. Four-channel machine, 12 locations to be tested, meant four times for each complete EKG; four times for you and the tech to go through these steps. When the test was over, they never, ever, wiped all the goop off you completely; you were left with a fair amount of this sticky gel still on you. Even at that age, it made me question the work ethic of the techs, although at that time, I don't think I would have been able to put it like that. And the techs never spoke to you except to tell you what to do and when to be still. Pleasantries were kept to the minimum. It wasn't that they were trying to be mean to you or that they didn't like children in general or even you. Also, I'm sure that the fact I was busy being a good boy, so much so that I literally almost never spoke even a single word, probably bolstered the impression that maybe there was no need for them to speak with me. But I think mostly it was just that I was a child. In those days they just didn't think that children felt or understood much. Logically, as they saw it, children really didn't need or require any sort of explanation of what was happening or being done to them. And so, they didn't.

9

After some time in the ICU, I was brought back to the ward, but I wasn't well. I was getting sicker and had no energy. *Lethargic* would be an apt descriptor, but it was worse than that. I lay pretty much motionless in bed all day. Things just weren't right.

They took blood for tests every morning and every night. Today, when you get a blood test, a phlebotomist, the name for the kind of tech who does the blood draw, taps a vein in either your hand or arm and takes several vials of the stuff at a time. Back then, they used something called a lancet. A lancet was a small piece of stainless steel roughly an inch and a half long and between three eights to half an inch wide. It had a V channel running down the center line that ended in an extremely sharp point. From the top view, it looked very similar to a child's paper airplane rendered in shiny metal. They didn't take the amounts they do today, they only needed a few drops back then. So, the phlebotomist would take one of your fingers and pierce it with the lancet. It didn't go in very deep, but still, you were being stabbed with the thing and it hurt enough that it wasn't something you'd look forward to. Worse, often the phlebotomist would have to stick you more than once to get the amount he or she needed because sometimes a stick wouldn't yield the amount desired, and sometimes no blood would come at all. That meant a second stick in the same finger or in a different finger altogether. The trouble was, every time they stuck you, your finger would heal in such a way that it made it more difficult to get blood the next time.

The phlebotomists came for the night draw after you were sleeping and would have to wake you up. One night, a male phlebotomist came to my bed and woke me for that night's draw. I remember him. He was a young man, maybe late twenties, good-looking, clean cut. He was very gentle, and he seemed to have a great amount of empathy for his patients. He spoke softly to me, handled me with careful tenderness. I don't know why this is, but in a lifetime of hospitalizations, it's been my experience that whether it was a phlebotomist or a nurse, the males were almost always gentler than the females. I think it's because the men know they aren't naturally as gentle as the females, and they're more conscientious about how they handle their patients. I could be wrong, but that's my theory. I'll give you an example of what I mean from this same timeframe.

One night, while sleeping soundly, a female nurse, (I don't remember ever seeing a male nurse back then) had to wake me to give me a pill. Apparently, she had trouble waking me. She took her flashlight, (the nurses all carried silver metal flashlights) and tapped me on the forehead with it until I woke. It was far from a gentle experience, and while she didn't hurt me outright, I remember I had to rub my forehead when she left. Oh, the pill she had to give me? According to her, it was something to make me sleep. To this day I can't figure that one out. Of course, it could have been something else entirely, but that was what she told me.

Anyway, this compassionate young man was seated next to me, prepared a lancet and sticks me. No blood. He sticks me again. No blood. He changes fingers. No blood. He's visibly upset. He knows this is hurting me. I never said a word the whole time, not even "ouch." I think that upset him even more. What he didn't know was that I had gone to my cave by the third stick. When all was said and done, he'd stuck all ten of my fingers multiple times and still hadn't gotten a single drop of blood for all his efforts. His concern for me was palpable, and he was upset by the whole situation. He kept apologizing to me, each apology a little more frantic than the last. He kept trying to comfort me, too, but still, he couldn't draw any blood. Finally, frustrated and deeply concerned for the harm he felt he was doing to me, he apologized again and left to get some help. By this time, I was fully in my cave, completely disassociated with what was going on. He came back with another person, but I don't remember them at all, not even if they were male or female, but I would bet the person was female. The fact was that I was deep in my cave by now, I could no longer see out of it. All of my fingertips had little band aids on them and whoever he had brought back with him made the decision that they would move down to the pad of one of my fingers. That would hurt a lot more than the tip, but really, what else could they do? So, they stuck me in this more painful place and successfully drew the blood they needed. For days after, they drew blood from my finger pads until they were able again to use the tips. You wouldn't believe how much that hurts or how it throbs for days.

That poor phlebotomist. I think that really shook him. I think the fact that I hadn't said a word, not a single word throughout the ordeal, somehow made it worse for him. My fingers were throbbing by the time it was over. I think he knew it, and it hurt him to think he had hurt me. But it wasn't his fault, and, oddly, I remember him as one of the nicest people during my stay there. A lot of people had been nice to me, but in my mind, he stands out.

10

Ten days after the X-ray, my condition hadn't improved, and I was continuing to deteriorate. Another X-ray revealed the fluid build-up had gotten worse. The decision was made that I had to be "double-tapped." This meant that the doctors wanted to drain the fluid from my chest. To do so, they had to "tap" me, as if I was now some maple tree in Vermont being forced to give up its sap. So, again I went for an operation, and this time they inserted a tube between my ribs on either side of my chest wall. It's no wonder that my impression of my stay at St. Francis was a series of operations. It was. When I woke from that one I was again in a different room and not under an oxygen tent. As it was when I had come to from heart surgery, that bed was tilted in a semi-reclined position, but this time, my position in the bed was more upright, closer to that of a seated position.

I could clearly hear the noise of a machine. I looked down to my left and discovered the tube, a big one, snaking out from under my blankets and followed it to the source of the noise. It was a machine, a pump, that looked a lot like one of those big, round room humidifiers with an equal in diameter, round glass container on top that was attached to the pump immediately below it. In the jar was the fluid that was being pumped out of my chest. It looked dark brown in color and it was thick and viscous. I heard the same noise to the right of me and, sure enough, there was another tube. At the time, the word *hose* seemed more appropriate, as it was nearly an inch round, attached to another identical machine, partially filled with the same vile-looking material as the other. I remember looking at these jars and thinking, *ugly jars of me.* Ugly jars of me. I still can't think of a better way to describe it.

At some point, a pudgy, middle-aged nurse in her white uniform and white nurse's cap came over to me. First thing she did was sit me up higher, as the angle of the bed was such that I couldn't help but obey the laws of gravity and kept sliding down, leaving me at less than the angle than was desired. She had to do this often. I remember her, can still see her face, her short curly brown hair that seemed to dare her nurse's cap to stay in place. It did; hair pins, I guess. I also remember her as kind but not particularly talkative.

Other than keeping me sitting in the right position, she had another task as it concerned me. She came over, holding a tube. Although I never saw what it was attached to, I was soon to learn it was a suction tube, and she asked me to cough. Cough? I didn't have to cough. She told me I had to and to give it a try, because if I didn't cough, and cough well enough, she would have to use this tube and neither one of us wanted that. We didn't? "Try," she said. I tried and made a couple of weak little coughs. You have to remember my chest had recently been split open and the smallest movements on my part were a cause for a great deal of pain. No, not moving at all, and certainly not coughing in particular, seemed to be in my best interest. Or so I thought. "Try harder," she goaded me gently. I tried but didn't do much better. Finally, she told me she would have to use the tube and had me put my head back and open my mouth wide. She put the tube in deep. Of course, it choked me, panicked me, but she kept that tube in, all the time it making disgusting sucking sounds, all the time me wishing it was over, all that time gagging, my chest on fire. When it finally was over, my throat hurt, and I was coughing just from the gag reflex. My chest was pounding with pain.

My parents came that night and my mother and I worked on getting me to cough "productively." But I still hadn't learned. It was incredibly painful. The next day the nurse was back with her suction tube. As in the day before, she had to suction me several times because I couldn't cough well enough to bring up fluid on my own.

The second night there was a nurse who was one of those exceptions, a bad exception, that every profession has. She was nasty. All she wanted to do was sit in her chair that was diagonally across from my bed. She didn't want to get up from it, and she didn't want to tend to me. I believe she was a private nurse, under my parents' direct employment. But gravity was still at work, and I kept sliding down on the bed. Each time she had to reposition me she got more annoyed, more frustrated. By the middle of the night she was being pretty rough with me, grabbing me hard and yanking me back to position. She took it as a personal offense each time I slid down, as if I was doing it deliberately just to inconvenience her and disturb her rest. By the middle of the night I was frightened of her. She didn't seem to be aware I just had major open-heart surgery, that my chest still felt like a truck had hit it. Or that I had two groin incisions, let alone that I had tubes coming out from either side of my chest. It was a long night.

But by the next day I had learned to cough productively. The kind day nurse was pleased she didn't have to put me through any more suction ordeals. That night I told my mother about the nurse from the previous night. If she had been a character in a cartoon, steam would have come out of her ears. She and my father left the room in an angry rush. I don't know what happened, or who my parents spoke to, but that night I had a different nurse, and I never saw the other one again.

But it wasn't all for nothing. I can still cough a very deep cough at will. I can scare you with it. I can make it sound deep. You'd think I was bringing up a lung. For years this skill served me well. It always surprised me that my parents, who had taught me how to cough that way, never caught on. All that mattered to me, however, was that it kept me out of school whenever I didn't want to go on any particular day.

11

I can't be sure exactly how much time I spent in that room attached to those machines, but at some point I was once again brought to an operating room. An X-ray had shown that the fluid had indeed been extracted and it was time to remove me from the pumps and to remove the hoses from me. The doctors were pleased with my progress, and I was returned to the large ward where my stay at St. Francis had started.

It had to be around this time that the first of my stitches had to be removed. I know I went home with stitches, most likely the ones on the sides of my chest for the pumps, but the stitches in my groin had to come out, and the stitches that had closed my chest were soon to follow.

In the fifties, they didn't have subcutaneous (under the skin) stitches made of materials that dissolved on their own and that left relatively small, thin scars. Doctors simply made a loop for each closure, one after the other, spaced evenly the length of the incision. You got used to the feeling of the stitches after a while, but they were irritating. A doctor, accompanied by a nurse, lifted each stitch at the knot with a pair of tweezers, and then with the aid of a small, sharp scissor, cut the stitch just below the knot. The area would, of course, still be tender, and the doctors were careful about how much pressure they used to lift the knot. I wouldn't say that it hurt exactly, but it did get your attention. When the scissors cut a suture, the skin would immediately fall back into place, relieving both the pressure made from the pull of the tweezers and the pressure of the suture itself. Then the most remarkable thing happened: the doctor, still holding the end of the stitch in his tweezers, gently pulled the catgut suture out. As the material made its way through the hole it had made, there was an almost sublime pleasure as it passed through. It felt sooo good as it was being pulled out. And once out, it was just, no other way to say it, a relief. A relief you almost didn't know you needed, but once discovered, had a way of giving your body what was, for all intents and purposes, a sigh. A giant, all-over sigh. It was wonderful. And when they were done removing the stitches from a particular incision, it would be a little sore from the recent manipulation, but overall you felt great. It quickly became that I looked forward to having my stitches taken out just because it felt good. Nothing, to this point, in this whole hospital experience had felt good, and, really, there shouldn't have been any expectation that it would. I took having my stitches removed as a gift, a brief respite from the boredom, pain and loneliness of daily life in the hospital.

12

At this point, the doctors were just giving me time to recuperate under their supervision. I have three powerful memories of this time. Two of them were small things that left a lasting impression, and one haunts me to this day.

I'm not sure of the timing of these memories and, really, it isn't important. The first occurred one night during visiting hours. My father picked me up, my butt sitting in the crook of his arm, my head higher than his, as he walked me up and down the other side of the ward. I had never been to that end of the ward and I got to see the distant neighbors for the first time. But that wasn't what made this moment special for me. It was the fact that I was with my daddy, and he was holding me, and I was proud he was my father and I was his son.

My father was the very definition of a "man's man." When he was young, he had been third runner-up for Mr. Universe in New York State. He played college football. He was in "The Golden Gloves." During the war, he killed at least one enemy in hand-to-hand combat. He was wounded by a U.S. naval barrage in a friendly-fire incident. He never spoke about the war to me except for the one time when he told me how he and a group of his buddies "borrowed" an army truck full of blankets while he was stationed in the Philippines, delivered them to an orphanage and then returned the truck without getting caught. When he told me this story, the one and only time he ever told me anything about the war, I was around twelve. He laughed as he remembered the prank and his buddies, but then the laughter stopped, and a cloud came over his face as some other memory superseded the orphanage story. What it was I'll never know, but the joy he had been experiencing just moments before drained from his face, and his features drew tight. He turned and walked away from me and continued to work on the lawn. In just the way that troubling memory was attached to my father's story, I have somehow attached the memory of him holding and walking me in St. Francis to the time he told me his war story. I loved my father, but I was somewhat of a disappointment to him. Born sickly, not any good in athletics, I was far from what my father wanted in a son. But I knew he loved me, and that day, as he walked me up and down the ward, both of us were proud and happy to be father and son.

The second memory happened one night during visiting hours. My parents told me they had a surprise for me. Just as it was that the time for visiting hours was strictly enforced, so, too, it was that children weren't allowed during visiting hours. So, my parents got me out of bed, walked me to the windows at the end of my side of the ward, pulled back the curtains and pointed. There, under a big tree, sitting on a green blanket were my two brothers and sister. When they saw me, they waved, and I waved back. As happy as I was to see them, and I truly was, I quickly became aware that there was something odd, even alien about the experience. Something was wrong. Then I felt it. A titanic shift in the continental plates that made up the geology of my world, the foundation of everything I had known to be true changed, changed forever in the violent earthquake that was happening right under my feet, right then, right at that very moment. A new paradigm had emerged, and it happened during those first few moments while I was waving to my siblings. It was easy for me to see, obvious, and yet I was sure I was the only one who saw it or understood it. As they waved happily, with Mom and Dad next to me, the whole family together as much as was possible at that moment, I saw something entirely new. This is what I saw: Peter, Michael and Neiani outside, enjoying a beautiful June evening, sitting on that blanket under that tree, and there I was, two stories up, in this building, this awful place where children across from you died, where ether and scars were given to me, where I had to lie still and not complain while scary and painful things were done to my body. I realized that it wasn't just a building and height that now separated us. No, it was something new, something that now separated all of us. I could see what it was clearly, see that they—and really, not even my parents standing right next to me—had any real clue as to what was going on in there, what was happening to me inside those walls, behind the glass and stone. And there it was, the disconnect. I had discovered the disconnect that had occurred between our two realities, and at that moment I was the only one that was fully aware of its existence. I understood that this disconnect would change everything forever. And in that moment, something else told me that for all my parents' visits, for all of their concern, and that of the doctors and nurses and nuns as well, that the bottom-line truth was that really, I was *alone*. I was doing this alone and it was up to *me* if I lived or died.

I suddenly understood that none of them would ever fully

understand what went on in there. How could they? All five of them would go home when visiting time was over, and I would still be in there. Their world, except for the absence of me, and the effects that my absence had on them all, was still largely intact; still familiar, still theirs. They would sleep in their own home, in their own beds, eat my mother's amazing cooking, wear their own clothes, have their own things, continue with their own lives, and most of all, they would all be *safe*. None of them were being stalked by death, but I was. I was in the fight for my life, and I knew it, had known it, knew it to my very core, and no member of my family, no one else at all, no one but me, could fight that battle. My family would go home, sleep, and when they woke none of them would see a sign that said NO FOOD hanging off the foot of their beds. They would never know what those two words had come to mean for me. They wouldn't be put under only to find out afterwards where they had been cut, cuts that would leave permanent scars, change their bodies forever. They wouldn't be wheeled away on a gurney multiple times, each time not knowing exactly what was going to be done to you, how it would feel when you came to, or even if you *would* come to at all. Seeing them down there did make me happy. I missed them, I missed them all terribly, but at the same time, it was at that moment I realized a shift had taken place and things would never be the same again. I was forever different. It was the first time I realized how different our lives had become, the first time I realized that things I had experienced had made a permanent river of separation between my life and theirs, and that there was no bridge and no map that would ever make it possible for us to be on the same side of the river again.

My mother once told a good friend of hers that the man she saw off to war, my father, never came back from that war; that the man who returned wasn't the man she had married. She had said that he was different, he had been changed. Well, I'd gone off to war, too, a different kind of war than my father's, but still a war, a war for survival, a war with battles and death. In war, you can see and experience terrible things, things that change you forever, things so horrifying that they ultimately affect the soldiers' families, too.

There, standing at that window at the age of five, I knew I would never be the same again, and that the family would never be the same again, either. As I stood at that window, waving to my siblings, I saw all this as clear as day. A tectonic shift of major proportions had taken place under the bedrock of the Taibbi family and things would never be as good as they had been just a few short weeks ago. And I also knew, also saw as clearly as day, *it was all my fault.*

13

My third memory is of Baby Carl. That's what I called him and my memories of him are the most powerful memories I have of all the time I spent at St. Francis. To this day, they are among the most powerful memories of my entire life. Carl was a baby in the ward whose bed was on the same side of the room as mine. His bed was against the wall just short of the windows where I had recently waved at my siblings. I loved Baby Carl, and during the time of my recuperation, the nuns had allowed me to visit him. I would climb out of my bed and run down the row of beds to play with--I'm guessing here now—the under-two-year-old baby. He might have been a little younger than that, but I do remember clearly that, as yet, he couldn't speak. For all I know, the reason for that might have been developmental, as he was a very sick child. Baby Carl loved to laugh, and nothing gave me more pleasure than to be the cause of that laughter. His laughter was infectious, and it made me laugh, too. Baby Carl's wide grin made everything all right again. The song of his laughter lit up my world. When we laughed together I was transported from inside those walls to a special place where nothing could hurt either of us. Laughter wasn't heard frequently inside of that ward, and I think the nuns enjoyed the sound of it as much as we did. I also think they thought we were good for each other because I was allowed to visit him several times a day. I couldn't wait for each visit. I remember dragging my parents down to meet him. Being that it was visiting hours, my parents and I met Baby Carl's parents, too. I went to play with Baby Carl while our parents spoke to each other in those hushed tones I'd grown accustomed to. The hushed tones meant that they were speaking of serious grown-up things, things we weren't supposed to hear or know about, things that meant they were talking about us. Usually I paid more attention to those types of conversations because I could generally glean so much from them. But that night I didn't care about any potential gleaning; I wanted to play with Baby Carl. Maybe I didn't want to hear what they were saying because I had gleaned enough already. His parents had that stricken look I'd seen recently on the faces of my own parents. They were younger than my parents. It seemed to me that my mother and father were trying to soothe them, trying to give reason for hope. One thing I knew, like me, Baby Carl was fighting for his life. It became that whenever my parents visited me they also visited Baby Carl's parents.

We had a game we used to play. Baby Carl had one of those toys, a nesting box, that was a box inside a box inside of a box, until you peeled all the layers away and you came to the surprise in the middle; in this case, a little toy bear. It wasn't really a box, it was tetrahedron, a ball made of little triangles, and in each triangle was the likeness of a smiling bear. The brown-colored bear in the middle was the embodiment of that likeness. The outer shell was baby blue, next was pink, but I don't remember any more from there. I would start with the toy fully assembled, and at the opening of each layer feign shocked surprise at finding another box beneath the last. As each of these layers were discovered, Baby Carl would laugh or giggle as if it was the first time he'd seen it, or my reaction to it. When we finally reached the toy bear in the center, and my surprise to this discovery was the biggest, Baby Carl would laugh so hard that his little arms and legs would swing and kick; his infectious laugh filled my heart with our mutual delight. I would then take all the pieces, duck down to the floor, out of his view, re-assemble the toy and Baby Carl and I would start the whole routine all over again, always with the same happy results. We never tired of the game.

Then one day the men with the gurney came and took Baby Carl. I knew they would be coming for him because my mother had warned me the previous night. I remember her warning me while wearing that very serious expression, an expression that had become like a code between us. She had communicated, and I had understood, that Baby Carl was in trouble. I watched him as the men with the gurney took him the next morning, passed my bed and went through the double doors across from me. I never really got a good look at him and we weren't able to make eye contact. As they took him, I watched with grave concern. I was worried, very worried, for my little friend.

It depended on whether you were having an *operation* or a *procedure* that determined if you would come back to the ward or not. If it was a procedure, you'd often come back to the ward the same day. If it was an operation, you went to recovery first. Baby Carl didn't come back that day. I kept praying he was in recovery. When visiting hours arrived along with my parents, I wanted to know if they knew. My parents had made friends with many of my doctors and because my mother was a nurse they seemed privy to a lot of what was going on. I could tell that they knew the answer; the first thing I asked my parents was if Baby Carl was all right. I was pretty sure I already knew the answer because Mother had that serious expression she wore when news was bad. She had come into the ward wearing it. No, she told me, he wasn't all right. He didn't make it, he was never coming back.

This news was a hammer blow for me. *He didn't make it? He wasn't coming back? He would never come back? Not Baby Carl, oh no, not him!* I don't remember anything else of that visit. I didn't go into my cave and I didn't cry either. I just went numb. It is not an exaggeration when I say that I never cried during the entire time of my stay in St. Francis, nor at anytime at all if it pertained to my heart problems. Not once, not a single tear, and not even for Baby Carl. I suppose in a way it could be argued that for me not to cry really meant I was in my cave to one degree or another, but I don't know. What I do know is that I loved Baby Carl. For a week or so he made life tolerable inside those walls. He had brought the only laughter, the only happiness that I had for that entire month, the month that seemed like a year. I missed Baby Carl. I missed him terribly then and I miss him still. But he does live on in me in as much as I can still see his happy grin, hear his laughter, see his arms and legs wave and kick in delight, see his face light up whenever we got all the way down to the toy bear. His laughter still warms me. I think of his parents, too. I remember the profound sadness each of their faces wore whenever I saw them. I wish I could see them now. I wish I could tell them how much I loved him or how much his gifts of laughter had meant to me; how his laughter was the only happiness I knew in that entire, dark time.

I wish.

And oddly, I wonder whatever happened to that toy.

Thank you, Baby Carl. Sleep well.

14

Finally, I was discharged, exactly 31 days from the day I
had been admitted, on July 9th, except only ten minutes
sooner, at 10:00 a.m. instead of the admission time of
10:10 a.m. I was leaving the hospital with a giant, hot pink
vertical scar on my chest that was already developing into the
huge keloid it would both become and remain for years to come,
with complimentary hot, keloid-becoming scars in both my
groins, both sides of my chest and various scars on my wrists, on
the insides of my elbows and ankles. But at last, I was going
home.

My parents had picked me up. Peter, Michael and Neiani
were waiting at home. I remember passing the Garden City train
station, the only landmark I recognized on the way to or from
the hospital and my home in Malvern. It had been a month since
I'd been in the big green and white Oldsmobile 98 sedan, or on
those roads or in my home. It all felt surreal. I had this strange
sense I no longer belonged in that car. I was still keenly aware of
the giant geological shift that had taken place that night by the

window, and how since that night nothing felt right to me any more when it came to me or the family, and, as I was to find out, it never would.

We finally arrived home. Neiani and Michael had greeted me as I came in. Peter was standing in the back hall, in direct line-of-sight with the front door. He was wearing black pants and a white dress shirt. Why he was wearing a white dress shirt, I don't know, but he was. I ran to Peter and threw my arms around him and hugged him tightly. My tears wet his shirt. Peter had been adopted at four and a half, after being bounced from one foster home to another. He had had a tough life before my parents made him one of their own, but some part of Peter had been hurt too badly before he came to us. He had trouble trusting in general and trusting that he really was a member of the family. But none of that mattered to me. All of them, as far as I was concerned, were my brothers and sister, and the lack of actual blood ties made no difference to me in the slightest. It never did, never has. Peter was my brother, my oldest brother, and I loved him, as I did Michael and Neiani. I don't know why my reaction with Peter was so powerful that day, but it was, and as I hugged him and my tears fell on his shirt, I remember he was surprised at my reaction to him and how he had difficulty with the idea of hugging me back, how my tears and reaction to him had startled him. He sort of put his arms around me, accompanied by a nervous laugh and a slight pulling back. He did his best, and his best was to pat my back with one hand as his other arm hung loosely around me. But that was okay with me, that was Peter. I didn't expect anything else, and it didn't matter anyway, because I knew that he loved me. Children know these things, sense these things and I knew that.

Somehow, hugging Peter made me feel like I was back in the house, but yet, not completely. Something was missing, and what was missing was any feeling of me—of me in that house. I had been gone too long and if I had been a dog, I would have thought that my scent was no longer there. I realized that I was home, but for some reason it no longer felt like home because my presence, my scent, was no longer there. I would have the same feeling again on the first day of camp. You knew you would be staying there, but everything was foreign, and it would take a while to get used to things. Nobody said it or acted in any way to convey what I felt, but I knew, and I think they knew, especially my siblings, that things were different. My family had been living there all this time without me and routines had changed and developed and none of the family routines involved me anymore. I felt like an intruder in my own home, and my own home no longer felt like home. I don't know if my parents sensed this feeling or not, but strangely, my mother walked me up the stairs to my bedroom, almost as if I was being shown where it was that I would sleep; almost as if I wouldn't know the way there myself.

It was when I entered my bedroom that all my fears were confirmed. The day I came home was a beautiful, clear July day. The sun was out and shining brightly. My room, with windows on two sides, was flooded with light, but it was no longer my room. The bright sun only added to this impression. Instead of being warm and welcoming, the light only accentuated what had changed. The room had been cleaned to such a degree that it had the appearance of being a spare bedroom, a guest bedroom, a bedroom no one lived in. All my stuff had been put away. I could see nothing of mine—no toys or clothes—nothing. The room was sterile. It looked like it had never been occupied before, and certainly like it had never been occupied by me. The bed looked like it had been made to pass army muster; the bedspread pulled so taut that if you bounced a quarter on it, the quarter would hit the ceiling. Pinned to the pillow was the relic of a saint, Padre Pio, that my mother had put there, and she showed this to me with great pride, convinced, I'm sure, that it had been at least partially responsible for my survival. Who knows? Maybe it had, but in any case, it didn't mitigate any of my feelings that that was no longer my room and that room was in a home that was no longer mine. But what confirmed those feelings the most was the smell. The room reeked with the unmistakable odor of disinfectants and cleaning agents. To me, it smelled a lot like the hospital. But worst, it no longer smelled like my room. There was no doubt about it, my world, my life and everything in it had changed, and it would never be the same again. When I went to bed that night, it felt like I was again sleeping in a strange place, in a strange bed, and more, I was still wishing for my things, the same things, and in the same way, as I had my first night in St. Francis. I wished I was in my own room again, the one that had been mine the night before I first left for the hospital. Finally, I rocked myself into an uneasy sleep, a stranger in my own home, a stranger in my own bed.

15

Of course, things were different. I was different, and that difference affected the entire family. Not only had the whole hospital experience changed me mentally, but physically, as well. I'd just been brought back from the precipice of death. Furthermore, I was frail and still in great danger, and I knew it. Remember, I'd been sent home with both the doctors and my parents knowing that the anomalous pulmonary venous drainage was still leaking and that the second ASD had not been repaired. I was far from out of the woods. I'd been sent home in the hopes that the area around the venous drainage would grow strong enough to tolerate a repair and that that tolerance would allow the second ASD repair to be made, as well. I was still walking that tightrope between life and death, and any wind could push me over to fall into the waiting abyss below. While I instinctively knew I was still in danger, my parents knew it for a fact. This must have been hell for both of them, but particularly for my mother. But the fact was, I still might not survive long enough before they could even attempt the repairs, and even if I did, odds were I wouldn't survive the operation.

The geologic shift I'd felt that night in St. Francis had radiated into the household, as I knew it would. The tectonic plates had shifted under our home, and the landscape had changed, and those changes presented themselves in multiple ways, some of which were quite surprising.

Mother had gone into full momma-bear mode, and I was the cub she was protecting. I became her focus to the extent that her protection over me came at the price of her almost ignoring the rest of the family. I got most of the attention, and understandable resentments from my father, Peter, Michael and Neiani began to build and my guilt started to grow exponentially as a result.

That fence my mother had started to build before my diagnosis, the one the rest of the family had to jump over if they wanted any access to her or me, had grown exponentially, as well. Now it was almost impossible for any of the family to get inside that fence, and worse, almost impossible for me to get out of. It wasn't until years later that I learned why my mother had been that way, but once I learned the reason, her actions became understandable, and they made me sad for her. I'll get into that part later. But for now and always, the Taibbi family had been divided into two very clear camps, and no one had any say in the formation of this family division except my mother. Now more than ever, the one thing I was certain of was that it was entirely my fault.

I don't know what my parents had told my siblings, not while I was in the hospital or while I was home. I don't know how much they knew, but I highly doubt they knew the whole story. Really, when you think about it, at that time Peter, the oldest, was nine, and the youngest, Neiani, was four, so what could you tell them at that age that would be understandable to them? But no matter, whatever sympathy or understanding they might have had was being mitigated by my mother's overindulgence towards me and their growing jealousy. From their point of view, and I find this completely understandable, my siblings never understood that I neither sought nor wanted my mother's overindulgence. I just wanted to be one of them, a brother in the family, a part of the gang. And, unfortunately, this was also becoming true of my father's attitude towards me. After all, it was his wife who had disappeared behind that fence. I was getting attention that rightfully belonged to him.

I don't really remember much about that year except for a few things. My parents had adopted a clever strategy for me. They didn't act like I was sick and wouldn't allow me to think of myself as sick. I was expected to do all the normal things for a boy my age. I was expected to act normally, too. That is, not to have an attitude of one who was sick or who had major heart surgery and was waiting for another. As grateful to them as I am for this, and I am, it became a two-edged sword. Even with that second edge, I'm convinced that this strategy helped keep me alive. It didn't give anyone in the family, especially me, a chance to wallow in all the negative aspects of the situation. It's possible, although I can't be certain, it gave me the impudence to develop a strategy of my own that I am certain saved my life in the long run.

Earlier, I stated that the tectonic shifts that reverberated throughout the family had manifested in some surprising ways, and what follows was the most surprising, which had a tremendous impact on me directly. I'd been discharged in early July, and while some time had passed, I do know it was still summer or towards the end of summer. Anyway, my mother asked me if I'd like to go to the beach and I excitedly said yes. I went to my room, got into my swimming trunks and was ready to go. Mom told me to put my beach jacket on and I did. I loved this jacket; I can see it so clearly in my mind that it might as well be hanging in my closet now. It was made of terrycloth; the back and front were black with white full-length sleeves. On the left breast, inside of a circle, was a yellow duck. This was why I loved this jacket as much as I did. The duck wasn't there just for decoration, if you pushed on it, it would quack! An article of clothing that was also a toy. Genius! So, with my little yellow beach bucket and matching shovel in hand, wearing my favorite jacket, my mother and I were off to Lido Beach, a section of Long Island's famous Jones Beach.

I recall it was a little cool at the beach and that we pretty much had the place to ourselves, most likely because it was during the workday and maybe also because it might have already been September. I was sitting on the beach, my jacket open, industriously shoveling sand into my yellow bucket and then pouring it onto a pile of sand I was trying to make into my own little sand dune. I wasn't sure what interested me more, making the hole in the sand or making the pile of sand. Of course, it didn't matter. I was happy. The day was beautiful, deep blue sky, dotted with big puffy clouds and soaring seagulls, a nice breeze, and the sound of the waves of the Atlantic Ocean breaking onto the beach adding the perfect soundtrack to a perfect day. Other people were there, just not nearby. I could see them down by the water's edge and hear them at play. For a little while, all that had just recently happened to me, the danger I was in, the family troubles, all drifted out of my thoughts, carried away and scattered by the breeze and dissolved into the sweet, salted air. The wind and the sun warming my face gave me a sense of peace. It was probably the first time I had felt that way since before it had been discovered that I was sick. For that wonderful moment, I was just a boy happily playing on the beach without a care in the world.

Then I noticed him. He was a young man, probably in his late twenties to early thirties, walking along the beach, coming right for us. As he neared me our eyes met, and I saw his gaze shift from my eyes to my chest. I watched as I saw his expression change from that of a guy just walking the beach, having his own good time and encountering a little boy and his mother on the beach to a sudden and startled expression. He was looking at my scar. He was the first person outside of my doctors and my family to see it, and his expression gave me my first feelings of shame and self-consciousness. You would've been startled too. It had become the keloid it had promised to be. It was literally about half an inch wide and the keloid made it about the same height. It was bubblegum pink, hot pink, rare roast beef pink, ugly pink. I turned to watch him as he altered his path directly to my mother, who was slightly behind me and to my right. Mom looked beautiful there on the beach, the wind playing with her hair, the breeze making her beach coat ruffle in the wind. And then it happened: that surprise, that moment that told me just how alone I was in this battle.

When he reached my mother, he pointed a finger at me, and these are exact quotes, said, "What happened to him?" Not missing a beat, my mother replied, "Oh, you wouldn't believe what I've been through!" And then my mother launched into her tale of woes to a perfect stranger, telling him about all the pain and misery *she* had been through because of my illness. To this day, I have never felt more invisible or of less substance.

Now, I know my mother didn't mean to hurt me, and certainly she had been through her own hell as well, but even at the age of five, her response to this stranger affected me as deeply as any one sentence uttered by another human ever has in my life, even till now. It struck me with the perception that for my own sake, I was never to complain. I was always to be stoic because there was no one interested in me or my story. It told me I was alone. My little heart was crushed as I listened to her talk. I needed to get away. I needed to get into my cave. But before I did, I looked up at the sky, almost directly above me, and I saw a seagull soaring in a tight circle, letting the thermal he was in lift him higher and higher, without him flapping his wings even once. He completely took my attention, and rather than go into my cave, I soared with him. The higher he went, the further and further away I got from my mother and the stranger. That seagull became my new cave and from then on I would alternate between him and my cave. He seemed to go up forever, still not flapping his wings, as he and I disappeared into a little dot in that beautiful blue sky. From the vantage point that I shared with that seagull, hundreds of feet above Lido Beach, I clearly saw that something had shifted as well in the relationship between my mother and me.

Aside from my mother and the seagull, there were several other outcomes that transpired that day at Lido Beach. From that point on, I didn't take off my shirt in front of anyone again for many years, except for family, and then eight years later with my friend Joe when we would go swimming together. Other than that, it wasn't until I was in my late teens, long after the keloid had finally resolved when I would again take my shirt off in front of not only strangers, but even people I knew outside of family.

And finally, that beach jacket that I loved so much took on a new and unfortunate association for me, and I never wore it again.

16

Time continued to pass, and I continued to grow weaker, but I tried to be a five-year-old who turned six during that year as best as I could. I had already finished kindergarten. Kindergarten was only for a half year and I'd finished mine before the diagnosis. While I don't remember it, I was beginning to have fainting spells, which put my parents and doctors on high alert. So, I had my second admission to St. Francis on August 24, 1959. The purpose of that visit was to determine exactly what was wrong and if I was strong enough for them to do anything about it. One thing was for sure though: After about 13 months of healing, I was doing poorly. So, on August 28, I had another cardiac catheterization. That one showed that the venous drainage was still leaking into my right lung, and that I had right ventricular and pulmonary hypertension. I still had the right-to-left shunt in the atrium, meaning I still had the other "hole in the heart," which, of course, they already knew. Bottom line: All of this had to be fixed and fixed *soon*.

I went home the next day, sporting two new scars in my groin, the smell of ether fresh in my memory, and with everyone, including myself, knowing that I was in more danger than ever.

17

I spent around a year and a half at home, I think to be given the chance to heal a little more before the second operation could take place. And as far as I know, I was still experiencing fainting spells. I did my best to be a normal six-year-old, running around the house and playing with my little sister, Neiani. In many ways, my parents' plan of refusing to treat me like I was sick or to allow me to think of myself as sick was working beautifully. Other than the fact that I was underweight for my age, there was really no outward sign that my life was in such a precarious spot. Earlier I stated that this line of thinking was probably what encouraged me to make an audacious strategy for myself, but when I think of it, really there were two. One I credit with giving me a better lifestyle and the other I credit with keeping me alive.

I was always a car nut—a *gear head*—and this was true for as long as I can remember. Also, since that encounter with the seagull at Lido Beach, I became a flying nut as well. Airplanes and cars were all I could think about. At the age of six I could identify any car on the road, make, model and year. When it came to flying, well, 1959 was part of the golden years of aviation. Chuck Yeager, who had broken the sound barrier less than ten years earlier, was a hero of mine and then Air Force test pilots were going faster than that. 1959 was the year the X-15 was introduced, the rocket plane whose test pilots took it to the edge of space, making them the first astronauts. I watched every newsreel on the subject of test flights and the myriad and fantastic aircraft coming out of the experimental programs of the day. If it was in *Life* magazine, *Look* or *Popular Science,* I was reading it, pouring over the pages, memorizing the photographs. If it was a movie or TV show that had something, anything, to do with flying, I was watching it. *The Spirit of St. Louis,* the story of the first airplane crossing the Atlantic non-stop, became my favorite movie. The fact that the flight had started just miles from my home or that the Garden City Hotel, the hotel one of my heroes, Charles Lindbergh, had stayed in the night before that historic flight, was a building I knew, and passed on my way to and from the hospital, only heightened my excitement for both the actual event as well as the movie. More importantly, it made the possibility of aviation for me to become a pilot someday more real as well.

My condition and my hospital stays had given me a great deal of time alone. Without realizing it, it had given me the time to learn how to think, and I thought often and hard about my situation. *I had been born with these crooked thumbs,* I had thought to myself long and hard, and my life had already become enough of a hell for me that I decided that the deformity would not add to it. I decided I would become dexterous enough with my crooked-thumb hands that they would never become an issue in my life. I was a weak child who didn't play sports, and I was already the kid that was made fun of, the one that attracted bullies and ridicule. My thumbs became the one place where I would draw the line, where I would not allow myself to be made fun of. I knew that meant my hands couldn't be a hindrance, that I couldn't be clumsy with them and that their ability to do things could never be an issue. So, I started building models: Models of cars, models of rockets and Air Force and Navy experimental aircraft. I couldn't build enough of them, and as time went on, the harder the better. Thankfully, my parents instinctively realized that there was something therapeutic for me in building them. I never told them the reason and they never asked, but they made sure I had a constant supply of them. Maybe it was because I built them skillfully—no gobs of glue, no broken parts—that made them know in their gut that those models were a good thing for me. So, I built them, and while doing so, taught my hands how to handle small parts and, at the same time, gain a delicate and precise touch, as well.

That strategy has served me well my whole life. It became that I love doing things with my hands. I became a car mechanic for a few years to help pay for college. I'm pretty handy around the house. I can do basic electrical work, basic plumbing and carpentry. If a fine necklace chain becomes knotted, I'm the guy who can untie it. And somehow, because of this pride I have at being more able than most with using my hands, I'm never embarrassed or self-conscious about others seeing them. I also think that because, at the most basic level in my psyche, my hands are such a non-issue that it also makes them a non-issue for all those that meet me, too. All this being said, however, there is still one circumstance where I am extremely self-conscious when it comes to my thumbs, and that is when people take my photograph. I don't like having my picture taken in the first place, but this only adds to my discomfort. There might be only a few photos in the world where my thumbs are visible, because whenever someone takes a photograph of me, I always hide them. Go figure.

The other strategy, the real one, the big one, I credit with saving my life. I call it, "bullying my heart." As I said, I was a kid who spent a lot of time by myself, and I occupied a great deal of that time just thinking. I may have only been six, but as it was even at five, I knew I was in grave danger. And, of course, I also knew that the danger was coming from inside of me, my heart. I guess I kind of took the attitude that my parents had taken, and act as if nothing was wrong and just build on that idea. I may not have known precisely what the problem was as I do today, but I did know that the problem was my heart. It was during this time between the operations that I developed this strategy and started to put it to use.

It wasn't really that big of a jump to go from having to act like I was okay to extending that premise to my heart. I was weak, I knew that, and while I don't remember the fainting spells, I do remember times when I'd be out of breath, my heart feeling "wrong" in my chest. At those times I would concentrate on my heart. I could feel it. I could feel its shape and exactly where it was in my chest. I would sit or lay down and tell it to get back to work, to stop being lazy. So, if I started to feel weak or out of breath, I would take a little time out and bully my heart and tell it to get back to work. Then, I would go back and continue the activity that made me feel weak in the first place, the whole time talking, sometimes yelling at my heart (internally, of course) to get going, to keep up, to stop being lazy. After not too long a while, I developed a friendship with my heart, a real and genuine friendship, and my heart and I opened a line of communication with each other. This is not an exaggeration; my heart and I became friends. As the years went on, I could rely on my friend to alert me whenever something was wrong. It also meant that nine times out of ten if a doctor told me *not* to do something then that would mean *I would have to do it.* For me not to would be an internal admission that I was sick, and that in my mind would tell my heart it was sick. I believed to the bottom of my soul that that would be the most dangerous thing I could do. Thinking like that, I was sure would put me in the grave. As years went on, this became a real sore point between me and my doctors, but I didn't care. I knew, *knew,* that to give in to a restriction would be the worst possible thing I could do. I *knew* it would be the death of me. And so, starting from the age of six, my heart and I were in constant communication with each other. And better still, our relationship blossomed, and we became best friends. That relationship lasted until I was forty-seven, when my friend having no more to give, and yet, still, with every last bit of life left in it, got me to the transplant and saved my life. I always likened my heart to a loyal German Shepherd who gladly gave its life to save its master.

18

By this time, I had started the first grade, but that was interrupted on October 18, 1959 by my third admission to St. Francis Hospital. This was the big one. I didn't go back to the same large ward where I was the first time I was there. This time I was put into a room with six beds. You had to walk down a long, narrow and twisty hallway to get to this room; it was really situated at the end of what would probably be called a breezeway on the second floor. There were only several small rooms in this part of the hospital, and they seemed to be set apart from all the others.

During my stay, I would occupy three of those beds at three different times, and I have distinctive memories of each. In that room, I got to wear pajamas, which was much more comfortable and a lot less shaming. We also had a little more freedom as I remember making friends with a boy who was in a glass-walled room at the edge of the breezeway. The room had glass on three sides and the glass started at about what would be chair-rail height to the ceiling. The hallway side was glass, as was the exterior wall. The wall that backed the headboard was also glass, as the room jutted out from the hospital and you had this marvelous 180-degree view of the hospital compound below. There were two rooms like that, one on either end of the breezeway, and I would soon be in the other one myself.

I would climb out of bed, make a left at the door, and walk the short distance to visit my friend. His name was Derrick. I remembered his name then the way I still do now. I knew that derricks were a type of crane and I just always associated his name with the crane that bears the same name. At the age of six I thought that was a very cool name. Still do. Derrick never got out of bed and our visits would constitute me standing beside his bed or hanging on the rails of his bed, and him sitting up slightly so he could see me better. We would talk and laugh, always having a good time together. Sometimes we just looked out the windows to the courtyard below and watched the doctors, nurses and nuns walking by, going from this building to that.

If I wasn't stealing a visit to Derrick, then just as in my last stay, I spent the day sitting in bed. This time, however, we were allowed to play with a very small assortment of toys supplied by our parents. I played with these toys on top of the over bed table. We didn't talk to each other too much in that room, mostly just staying to ourselves. I don't recall speaking with any of the children in that room. For that matter, I don't remember the room ever being full, either. But, as yet unbeknownst to me, trouble was brewing, and not with my heart, but between one of the nuns and my mother.

I don't know how it started but I would guess that somehow this nun—I don't know her name but we all called them "Mother," so that's how I'll refer to her—and my mother had a problem with each other. That wouldn't be too hard to fathom if for some reason this nun and my mother were in some disagreement about my care. My mother was still in full momma-bear mode, and it still wasn't wise for anyone to do something she didn't approve of. I think it was something on that order that caused the friction between these two. I remember a night when my mother and this nun were obviously having words. I was in my bed, last on the right in relation to the door, and they were in the doorway speaking in hushed, animated, angry tones. It was easy to see that my mother was mad; that both of them were mad. I still don't know what it was about. I don't know if it was about my care or the fact that I would visit Derrick or even something else, but whatever the subject of the conversation was, the confrontation left both women fuming.

The next day, I got my first hint of things to come. I was playing in my bed with my favorite and newest toy. It was a clear, egg-shaped acrylic dome set over a colorful base. Under the dome was a large pink, flower bud. There was a twisted rod with a wooden handle sticking out of the top of the dome. As you pushed down on the rod, it would make the floor the flower bud was sitting on spin. The rod was spring loaded, so it always returned to its original position. The idea was to push the rod up and down as fast as you could, and as you did, it would make enough speed that centrifugal force would open the bud and reveal the dancing prince and princess hidden inside. I loved playing with that toy. The mechanical nature of the twisted rod and how it spun the bud and the floor inside the dome gave me the perfect opportunity to watch the application of centrifugal force in action. This absolutely fascinated me. Besides, I loved seeing the princess. It was not usual for my father to approve of a toy with a pink flower bud for his son, but I also knew that he liked this toy, too. I figure he liked it for the same reason that I did. Flower bud or not, there was just something about the mechanical nature of this toy that was fascinating.

So, there I was, quietly playing with this toy, when Mother Nun and a young nun, a novice, one who I had never seen before, appeared in the doorway of my room. It quickly became apparent that they were looking at me and speaking about me. It was obvious that the looks I was getting from Mother Nun were not looks of approval. I couldn't hear all of what they said, but then—and this I heard clearly—Mother Nun slightly lifted her hand in my direction and said, "This one's a brat." As she said this the younger nun nodded solemnly. A *brat*? I couldn't believe my ears. I never said anything to anyone, except Derrick. I never complained, and I always did as I was told. I didn't even say "ouch" when something hurt, and that's not an exaggeration. Even at that age, though, I wouldn't have known what to call it, but I knew I was being slandered. I remember sitting there wondering what I could have done to deserve being called such a thing. Of course, now I understand I really wasn't the issue at all. What was really going on was that my mother and this nun didn't like each other one bit and Mother Nun was doing nothing more than projecting her feelings for my mother onto me. Little alarm bells went off in my head and I got nervous. Instinctively, I knew no good could come of this. I continued to play, but uneasily.

At this point, I want to say something about St. Francis Hospital. I owe my life to that hospital, my doctors, Dr. Mannix and Dr. Balboni, the nurses and nuns, and all the rest of those who helped me. They did everything they could to save my life, and that they did. They cared about me and they took care of me. While it's true that children were treated very differently in those days than they are today, that was nothing more than the convention of the day, common throughout society, hospital or not. My treatment as a patient was first rate, and frankly at that time, I doubt if any other hospital anywhere could have saved me, could have pulled off the medical miracle that Dr. Mannix and St. Francis did. Everyone there made sure that I was comfortable and was getting the care I needed. So, what I'm about to relay next I look at as an exception and certainly not the norm for the kind of care I received. Every profession has those in it, who for lack of a better term, is a *rotten apple*. I look at that encounter to be unique to this nun, to this one person in a hospital of hundreds of others who would never have done or condoned what happened next. In all these years, and even back then, I never confused this one nun with the hospital in general or all of the great caregivers St. Francis provided for me.

It was the middle of the night and I was sound asleep. When I say *middle of the night,* all I know is it was well past bedtime and the hospital had taken on that aura that only an institution well past regular business hours could take on; not quite dark and not quite quiet. I had no clock to reference to and it could just as easily have been midnight as it could have been four in the morning. All I know was that one moment I'm sound asleep and the next moment I'm being grabbed roughly. Mother Nun was doing the grabbing. I had been lying on my side, turned away from her and then she was taking hold of me, turning me onto my back. Of course, I was startled, and immediately frightened. She kept saying things like "wake-up you" and "get-up you." There was no kindness to be found in her actions or voice, and her face was creased with anger. Her anger terrified me, and the way she handled me confirmed my fears. She lifted me up against my will and plunked me down onto a cart with some sort of white cloth covering it. It wasn't a gurney, it was a cart like the kind nurses used to bring juice or milk to the children with. This is when I noticed the others. Behind Mother Nun were other nuns, four to six of them, and all of them were young. For all I know some or all were novices, but I can't be sure.

I was being wheeled down the hallway with one hand of Mother Nun holding me down at my chest as the other hand steered the cart. The other nuns fell in behind and to the side. I was panicked, and yelling, "Let me go, let me go!" While I'm crying, Mother Nun said things like, "This will teach you." "I'm going to show you." and "This will teach you a lesson." I can't remember everything she said, but I do remember hearing the word *brat* a number of times. I'm also of the impression she was speaking to the others as much as she was to me and to herself.

We finally reached our destination—a girl's bathroom. I found out what that room was just a few years ago when I visited the hospital on a nostalgia trip before the buildings I had occupied were all torn down to make way for new structures. Oddly enough, a friend of mine worked at St. Francis hospital and when I told her this story, she recognized the room from my description. She had been right, it was the same bathroom, a girls' bathroom, something I never knew, and it was a short distance down the hall from my room.

The lights were on, but not all of them, as most of the room remained in the dark. The whole room was covered in white tile. Around a corner and in the back was an area with a large shelf, also made of white tile. Mother Nun snatched me off the cart in a single, arch-like motion and plopped me down onto the cold, hard tile. In the blink of an eye, I was naked, naked in front of all of those women. I may have been six, and I may have been panicked, but I was also ashamed. My level of shame and embarrassment was overwhelming, and my terror had grown exponentially. Never in my whole experience at the hospital had anyone ever treated me in such a manner. No one in my life had ever treated me that way. I knew from the visible anger in her face, the twisted hatred that creased her old features, the tone in her voice, and the way she was handling me that it had nothing to do with my care or a procedure that had been order by a doctor. No—this was payback. This nun was going to teach me and my mother a lesson, and I was going to be the conduit of her revenge.

She spun me over, with me kicking and crying. Behind me was an I.V. pole, and hanging from it was an enema bag, made from that ubiquitous, red rubber. Attached to it was a long red, rubber hose. I knew what that meant. Mother Nun was directly in front of me and the shelf. The other nuns had now taken up position behind her. To me, none of them looked pleased at what was going on.

Mother Nun took the hose, and well, I doubt I have to say where she put it. I'll say this, even if she did everything during this incident with—how shall I say?—a less than delicate touch, she at least didn't deliberately hurt me during the insertion. Still, it was against my will and I was screaming, 'No, no, no! Don't do it. Stop. Stop!" But she didn't stop, and she wasn't gentle, but at least she didn't physically injure me.

I don't believe I'd ever had an enema before, but I knew what they were. Because we had a bag just like it in my home, I was familiar with the concept. Once the hose was, to put it delicately, "in position," Mother Nun released the clamp from the hose that was keeping its contents in the bag and a flood of cold fluid suddenly entered. It was nothing short of shocking. Call me a brat if you will, but I hadn't stop screaming that whole time and the dreadfully cold fluid certainly did nothing to calm me. It made me fight more, but Mother Nun kept a firm hand on my lower back and kept me planted on that shelf despite my kicking legs and flailing arms.

At the time, I wouldn't have believed it possible for the situation to get any worse, but suddenly it did. A new sensation started taking hold of me and a different kind of panic started to consume me. As this sensation grew, I started to scream more and more loudly. "Stop, stop, stop it," I pleaded. "I'm full. I'm full!" Still, she didn't stop. I looked over at the other nuns, and I could see from their faces that they were horrified at what was happening. I made eye contact with one of them. It was only for a moment, but I still remember what she looked like. We made eye contact for a brief second and then she turned her head away from me. In that short moment, I saw that her face was burning with a shame of her own. I'll never forget her or that expression, but it gave me a small degree of comfort. Mother Nun continued to ignore my pleas. I started screaming, "I'm going to explode! I'm going to explode!" She continued to ignore me.

And then I did.

The hose blasted out of me violently, followed by what could only be described as my own personal geyser. Fluid shot out of me at hypersonic speed and Mother Nun became the recipient of my own exploding "oil well." It hit her in the face, landed all over her habit, as well as on me and the shelf. For the first time during this event, I wasn't the only one screaming. Mother Nun let out her own shriek of horror. I looked up and saw that the other nuns were both disgusted, and at the same time, reluctantly amused, their heads bent, and their hands covering their mouths to hide their involuntary giggles.

This turn of events enraged Mother Nun, and for the first time, she let go of me to wipe her face in disgust and anger. I know that part of the story sounds funny, and retribution can be a wonderful thing, and even though it registered somewhere deep in my mind that she got *hers*, at the time it didn't mitigate any of the terror I was experiencing. Not only was I naked in front of all of those strange women, but I was covered in my own feces to boot. My shame only became greater as did my fear of

Mother Nun, who now had even more reason to be angry with me.

Despite my fears to the contrary, that new development did not escalate the situation. Next thing I knew, she was wiping me off and putting my pajamas back on. I'm not even certain if I was washed. By that time, I had become completely traumatized and reduced to a sobbing ball of jelly. At least, I thought to myself, the worst was over. The thought didn't placate me, though, as I continued to sob uncontrollably. Deep, painful sobs that rattled me all the way to the center of my being. I was placed back on the cart, again roughly, rolled back to my room and unceremoniously put back to bed.

For some reason, that night, I was unable to find my cave or fly with my seagull. I just lay in my bed in the fetal position, weeping and rocking. I finally fell asleep. The next day I told my parents what had happened, and I swear to you, fire shot from my mother's eyes while at the same time my father's face distorted under the building pressure of cold, stone anger. My parents were enraged. They left the room in a determined fury. I don't know what happened, I don't know who my parents spoke to. I'm not even sure if I ever saw Mother Nun again or not. It didn't matter. It was too late. Nothing could undo it. Nothing ever has. And once again the whole world would be different for me forever. *I* would be different forever. Something inside of me had been broken, snapped and from that night all the way to now, I never felt completely safe again.

19

Some days have passed and I'm in the same room, but for some reason I'm no longer in the same bed. Now I occupy the first bed to the immediate right of the door as you enter. I am no longer visiting Derrick. I don't remember why, but my best guess would be because he was no longer there. I don't know where he went or why, just that one day he was gone. I know I was never told to stop visiting him, so that couldn't be the reason. I seem to remember it being a bright day, but why I thought that I'm not sure because my room had no windows. But what I do know is that this was the day before my next and most dangerous operation.

I was lying in bed when a young, dark-haired, handsome priest walked into the room and over to the right side of my bed. He was carrying a small box, which he placed on the bed stand next to me. His name was Father Grappone and even though he was smiling and being very pleasant, underneath his smiling guise he was wearing the face of a man with an unpleasant task to perform. Father Grappone was a gentle, sweet man and he was there to administer, as it is commonly called, Last Rites, or, as it's properly called, the Anointing of the Sick. Six years-old or not, if you're raised as a Catholic in an Italian household, you know what Last Rites are. They are the Sacrament that is given to those who are either dying or about to die or who could die in the very near future. As part of Last Rites, the person is given a chance to renounce their sins through confession and receive the Sacrament of Absolution and have their sins forgiven. In the Catholic Church, a child below the age of seven who has yet to receive their First Holy Communion, the Sacrament of being able to receive the Body of Christ symbolically through a wafer (the Eucharist) is considered innocent. Therefore, I wouldn't have to make a confession and do penance; nor would I receive the Eucharist. But I could receive the blessings and be anointed with the Holy Oils.

No one had to tell me how dangerous the next day was going to be for me. The condition I had was often fatal to the children who had it. When I survived my first operation, I had beaten 50/50 odds. So far, so good. But I needed a second operation, not only to close the second hole, but also to solve the anomalous pulmonary venous drainage. To this point, *no one had survived two open-heart operations to fix holes in the heart before,* let alone the added plumbing repair. I was in it deep!

It's funny, no one told me how dangerous the operation was going to be, but I knew anyway because in so many unintentional ways, I *had* been told. The message was sent to me in the expressions my parents wore as the day of the operation grew closer and closer. Oh, my parents tried not to show their fears, but I could read them; I knew. I was told by the tenor that those hushed conversations between my parents and the doctors had taken on. I could hear the fear and the urgency that they contained. And now, if I had any doubts before, a priest showing up at my bedside told me everything I needed to know. After all, I didn't receive Last Rites for the first operation, had I? Death was stalking me, and I was about to go into battle. That was why Father Grappone was there and, as I said, I knew it. But I couldn't allow myself to think of him as real. I couldn't allow myself to think of him as a priest administering Last Rites. It was the last thing I needed in my mental preparation for what lay ahead. This one would have to be handled differently. I didn't go to my cave, or fly with my seagull; instead, I used laughter.

In a very serious and deliberate way, Father Grappone opened his box and took out his stole and put it on. The stole is a scarf-like vestment, a narrow band of decorated cloth that hangs down from the neck and covers both breasts. It signifies patience. Next, he took out his little jars of oils.

I was watching all of this, but smiling and acting as if this was just a friendly visit. I knew what he was doing and about to do but I couldn't give in to it. I think all of this made it much harder for the Father. The more I smiled and laughed, the more serious he became. There was a part of me that wanted to accept what he was doing, (see, Mom, I *did* pay attention in Catechism classes) understood what he was doing, but I didn't dare give in.

Father was praying over me and then started to bless me with the oils. To do so, the priest dipped his thumb in the little urn that contains the oil and then blessed me while making small signs of the cross on my forehead and chest with the oil. It was at this point that I started to giggle, especially when he crossed my chest. It tickled a little and I allowed that to become light laughter. I almost had to force it a little. I believe it was my laughing that did the poor priest in, because he had tears running down his cheeks and was fighting for his composure. I knew what was going on. I knew what his tears meant. I knew that from his perspective he was giving Last Rites to a child who would most

likely die the next day. I knew that he thought I was some innocent who didn't understand the gravity of his situation or what
Last Rites were about. I knew that the way I was acting was
terrible for Father Grappone, and that it was making his job
harder, tougher, and more emotional than it would have had to
be. I knew all of this. But I also knew I needed to be in a certain
state for the morning. I knew I had to be prepared for battle.
Don't ask me how I knew all of this, I just did. Best I could say
was it was instinctive. I just somehow knew it, knew it down to
the deepest part of my soul. I knew I couldn't even *think* of the
idea that dying could become a reality. I knew I couldn't let the
tiniest sliver of the thought of death—my death—take the
slightest hold in my mind. Like I said, I knew I had to do it for
my survival.

When he was done, he ceremoniously removed his stole and
packed up his little box. He left the room with his shoulders
bent, head down, and tears streaming from his eyes. I felt badly
for him; I wish I could apologize to him now. But I had to do
what I had to do and that was that. Sorry, Father.

20

As it has happened for eons, and will continue to do for eons more, the next day came: October 29, 1959. Oddly, I don't remember them coming for me, I don't remember the gurney ride to the OR. I remember the anesthesia mask and the hand that held it filling my sight once again and the horrible smell that went along with it, but compared to my first surgery, I don't remember nearly as much. I think in today's terms it could be said I don't remember as much because mentally I was, "in the zone."

But I do remember something else, something quite different, and I remember it vividly. The operation was in full swing, my chest was cracked open and rib spreaders are keeping it open. Of course, this I only know intellectually because I was knocked out at the time. But then something happened that I remember in great detail. Suddenly, my eyes are opened. I see a circle of doctors hovering over me, their masked faces showing eyes and foreheads knitted in concern under their surgical caps. Their voices are quiet but intense. After a few moments of this, I floated over to the top of a cabinet on the other side of the room, on my right side as I lay there. I could still see the doctors in their circle, but now from the perspective of my new vantage point. I remember thinking I must look like a little monkey sitting up here. I could see everything: the whole room, the full length of the table with me on it, the large, circular light above the table, the heart-lung machine, the little table holding the surgical instruments—everything.

Next thing I know, starting from a position above my feet as they lay on the table, the ceiling is split by the most beautiful shaft of light. It didn't look like a single shaft of light, but more like an array of beams like those you see occasionally breaking though the clouds on a summer's day. It was bright and, yet, at the same time it was soft and soothing. The light wasn't white and it wasn't silver, but it was breathtaking in its beauty and had a shimmering quality to it. The doctors didn't seem to notice the light but just kept on working. The shaft grew larger and larger, and up where the ceiling used to be higher, puffy white and silvery clouds had formed. The surgical light above the table and the ceiling were consumed by the clouds. Then, a face formed, beaming and smiling down at me. It was the face of a kindly old man with long white hair and a long white beard. He smiled warmly at me. It made me feel good. Other clouds now formed a staircase from my open chest to the clouds above and ultimately to that beatific face. From my perch on top of the cabinet, I watched as I saw myself get up out of myself from the table, wearing a long, flowing, white robe. I was carrying a white harp with gold strings and I started to slowly ascend the staircase. I got about three-quarters of the way up. Then, in the next moment, I looked up from the table again at the circle of doctors above me, and just as suddenly as it had started, it was over. The memory ended there.

Think of this what you will, but I went into the operation without this memory and came out of the operation with it. This memory has never changed; never diminished. A while ago, partly as research for this book and mostly just to see him again, I visited Dr. Balboni and his wife Mary at their home. He was my cardiologist while Dr. Mannix was my surgeon. I told him about this incident and he told me that I had the physical details of the room correct. Was this an out-of-body experience? I believe so. I think we see God the way we see him in our minds, in the way that He is real for each of us, and the way I saw Him that day certainly fits the description of God as a six-year-old Catholic would see Him.

Some time after I was home—two months, a year, two years, I don't remember—my mother told me that she had been told by the doctors that I had died while on the table. I heard her repeat that to many people, many different times over the years. When she first told me that, my thoughts immediately went to this memory and it finally made sense. I never told my mother of that incident and never told anyone of it at all until many years later.

Believe it or not. I'll let you be the judge on this one.

One thing, however, *is* certain: During that operation, a miracle *was* performed. Dr. Mannix had the daunting task of not only closing the second hole but also of correcting the plumbing problem. He had the brilliant idea of cutting my heart where the anomalous pulmonary vein was and folding it over my heart to give the vein a strong attachment point. He did this and fixed the other hole, and, for the first time in my life, made my heart whole. With this ingenious remedy, he both saved my life and made me the first person to survive two open hearts for IASD repair.

Once again, I woke up under an oxygen tent, but this time feeling much worse than I did after my first open heart operation. Again, I felt like I had been run over by a truck, a bigger truck this time; and to say that I *woke up* is not quite accurate. As before, anvils were holding my eyelids down and the pain in my chest was absolutely crushing. When you're in that much pain it's hard to localize it. *When you're in that much pain* your entire body is wracked with it. *When you're in that much pain* even the hairs on your arms hurt. All I can say is that it must have been one mother of a truck that hit me. My head throbbed with an anesthesia-induced headache that threatened to split my skull open with its clanging hammers. The fog of anesthesia was thick, almost impenetrable. I have always found it difficult to come back from anesthesia. It's much easier, much more comfortable, to just drift back with the anesthesia to this place under the comforting sea, this place beneath reality, where you have no thoughts, no pain, and no existence. My mother was holding my hand under the oxygen tent, as I knew she would be, but she hadn't noticed that I had come to, to whatever degree of coming to I had. We were next to a window and again the plastic was barely translucent, thus everything I saw was distorted by both the plastic and the sun shining from behind her. My mother was quietly saying part of a little Italian phrase we said to each other. She would say, "Figlio beddo," roughly translated Sicilian for "My beautiful boy," and I would answer, "E tu ma" or "You're my mother." I don't remember how many times she said it. For all I know, that might have been the only time. But I heard it, and gathering all the strength I had, I answered weakly, "E tu ma."

As she sat in her chair, holding my hand, Mom made a little

jump that was accompanied by a small gasp and then she bent down and put her forehead against the plastic where my hand was and broke down crying. She said it again and I again answered her. She said something to my father, who I couldn't see as she continued to cry. I think I registered movement from him, but I can't be sure because a moment later I had allowed myself to be pulled back under, deep beneath the comforting sea.

21

S ome days have passed. How many, I'm not sure, and I'm in a different room feeling much better. I'm not in too much pain. I suspect painkillers have something to do with that. But I'm alert and improving. I think I was in what they call a step-down room, a place you go when you are no longer in, as it was called then, ICU, or Intensive Care Unit, but are not yet well enough to go back to your regular room. I don't think I was there for too many days.

Unlike any of the other rooms that I can remember, except ICU, I was alone in this room. There was a privacy curtain pulled halfway around the bed and there was a window to my right, somewhat above me. I couldn't see out of the window, but it let in a lot of light, something I always found comforting.

Just then a doctor marched in accompanied by an entourage of six medical students. I can still see them clearly enough in my mind that I can count heads. I'd never seen that doctor before. He was of medium height and build and had salt and pepper hair with a neatly trimmed beard to match. I'd say his hair was a little more salt than pepper. As he entered, he abruptly pulled the curtain back and made his way to the foot of my bed to retrieve my chart from its holder on the footboard while the students took positions on the left side of the bed. They came within a foot of the bedrails, which were, of course, up. He came over to the other side and lowered the railing. He never said hello or anything to me at all. He pulled the blankets off me with one quick motion. A moment later his hand was under my back and he lifted me into a sitting position. Once I was in position, he untied my hospital gown, lifted it off me and lay me back down flat on the bed. The only thing I remember him saying was, "Now this is an interesting case," as he flipped through my chart. From the time he came into my room to the time I was naked couldn't have even been 20 seconds.

I didn't move, didn't say a word. I almost never spoke in the hospital to anyone except my parents, Baby Carl, or Derrick. The doctors and the nuns had to be satisfied with one or two-word responses. Remember when they had to double-tap my chest and drain the fluid after the first operation? The doctors didn't know anything was wrong until my temperature went through the roof. The double-tap was the response to a serious infection, and until they cleared my lungs and the infection, I was in jeopardy. The doctors wanted to know why I hadn't complained and they instructed my parents to tell me not to be so stoic, that I had to let them know if something hurt me. But things often hurt, and I had been instructed to be a good boy and not complain. Somehow it had just become easier to never say anything and instead climb into my cave whenever I needed to.

And again, I didn't say anything or do anything, but never-theless, I was both mortified and horrified. One moment I was lying by myself and the next I was naked in front of seven strangers. In those days it wasn't commonly thought that children that age were capable of feeling shame and other similar emotions, but, of course, they are capable of such feelings, and to a great extent. In the matter of a few seconds any feelings of safety, modesty, and, most of all, dignity, were torn away from me along with my gown. But worse, my new condition put me in a state of complete and utter powerlessness. Beyond the shame and embarrassment of my sudden nudity, that feeling of absolute helplessness was overpowering and terrifying. What was I to do? I didn't even know where to look, where even to put my eyes. All I knew was I didn't want to be any part of that situation. I certainly didn't want to look at the doctor anymore, so I slowly turned my head toward the students. Maybe that was worse. There were five men and one woman standing in two rows of three. The men were very intent on what the doctor was saying to them; a couple of them were taking notes, the rest were looking at my naked body in earnest, almost as if they thought the intensity of their gaze would get them a better grade; all except for the female student. She was a tall blonde with a pageboy haircut standing in the second row on the right. She was thin and taller than most of the others. Most of all, she was the only one there who was truly looking at *me*. She saw what was going on, she saw I was deeply embarrassed, ashamed and frightened. Of all seven of them standing around my bed staring down at me, including the doctor, she was the only one who was looking at the *patient* and not a slab of biological meat, not something that was just an "interesting case." She, God bless her, saw the little boy in that bed; *she saw me.*

Our eyes caught for the briefest of moments and her empathy, her feelings towards me and the situation we both found ourselves in, was obvious. She looked sad herself, and I could tell the circumstance disturbed her. I could recognize her today if I were shown a photo of her from back then. I wonder if she ever said anything to the others about my treatment. I don't think it would have mattered if she did. That was the way it was back then. Thank God, there were exceptions, like Dr. Mannix and Dr. Balboni. They spoke to me during an exam and let me know what they were going to do and asked if it would be all right. But again, they were the exceptions, at least as I experienced it. I'm sure either of them would have done something to protect my dignity in the same situation; it would have mattered to them.

And, I could tell, it mattered to *her*. Sometimes when I think of this incident, I hopefully imagine that it had an effect on her and the way she ultimately practiced medicine. I like to imagine it had an effect that made her a better and more compassionate doctor than she already would have been. I allow the thought to comfort me, to believe that my pain that day would at least not have been for nothing and that it somehow helped others down the line. Silly, huh?

After just a few moments of eye contact, I turned my head from her kind and compassionate face and looked upwards. I took myself back to that day at the beach with my mother. I could see the brilliant blue sky over Lido Beach, and there against a backdrop of clouds was my seagull, slowly wheeling in a thermal. For the first time in the hospital I chose to ride with him instead of crawling into my cave. So, I rose from my place on the bed, until I was high, high above, no longer visible to the doctor and students far below. I could see the doctor discussing my case with his students, but I couldn't hear a word he was saying because I was too far away to hear anything anymore. After a while I saw the doctor, again without saying a word to me, put my gown back on me, put the bedrail up, and partially redrew the curtain and leave with his students in trail. As for me, I continued to fly with my seagull for a long time afterwards, lazily circling the sky, riding the thermals high up in the deep blue heavens where no one else could find, see or touch me. It was a long time before I returned to earth and the bed where my body lay.

22

It's funny to me how much I both remember and, at the same time, don't remember, of my second operation. I remember my mother responding to me in the ICU, but I don't remember much else that happened in that room. I remember the doctor with the students in the step-down room, but not much else. I don't remember how I got from the ICU to there and, again, I don't remember going from the step-down room to where I ended up next, which was the other of the two little glass rooms overlooking the courtyard, the other of which had once held my friend Derrick. These rooms were very small, barely able to contain the hospital bed I lay in, and unlike Derrick, who had me to visit him from time to time, I had no such visitors. It was back to the same routine of being completely alone for the entire day, except for the occasional ministrations of the nurses, nuns, doctors, and, of course, my parents' visits. But I don't remember any of those visits, except a small part of one of them. I just know intellectually that the aforementioned had to have come into the room at some points during the day.

But I do remember the gift my first-grade class gave me that had to have been delivered to me by my parents, which is the one visit I partially remember. It was a class project. What the purpose of the project was exactly, I don't have a clue. I do know that every student was given a little square pot with a couple of cotton plants growing in them. What my classmates were instructed to do with them is still a mystery to me. I do know that a couple of cotton plants planted in actual dirt would never be allowed in a modern hospital for fear of what kind of bacteria could be lurking in the soil, but I got my cotton plants and they were placed on the windowsill right behind my head.

I was fascinated with these plants; both by how prickly they were and, yet, how at the same time they had little tufts of soft cotton clinging to them. The contrast that the plants could be prickly and soft at the same time enthralled me. Beyond that, my imagination went wild with the idea that I could cultivate them into an entire crop and that I could become a rich cotton baron. This idea was very exciting to me. Even though it hurt to turn on my side to look at them, I stared at these little plants for large chunks of the day. I envisioned great fields of cotton, as far as the eye could see, all begotten from these few plants. I daydreamed how successful they would make me. With these little cotton plants I would become *Steven, the Six Year Old Cotton King*. Hey, if you were alone as much as I was when I was a child, your imagination would've become pretty active, too. My imagination became my magic carpet of adventure and escape.

Then, the next thing I knew, I was back in my room across the hall where this particular trip to the hospital had started. Again, I have no recollection of changing rooms, nor what happened to those plants with which I was going to build my dynasty. All I know is that they didn't make the trip across the hall with me or follow me home.

Even though I was again in the same room, I was now in my third bed. This time I was in the middle bed on the left side of the room as you looked in. As I said before, Mother Nun wasn't there anymore, and I found a small sense of safety knowing I would no longer have to deal with her in any way. But I had a nickname given to me by another nun. Who she was, I don't know, but once she named me, all the nuns started calling me by the nickname, too. The name she gave me was "The Crooked Cross." They called me that because the incision for the second operation was horizontal instead of vertical. The incision started almost under my arm, just below one breast, followed the lower contour of the breast, went straight across my chest and then followed the lower contour of my other breast ending just short of under my other arm. Since I was the first to survive two open-heart operations for this kind of a repair, I was also the first to have scars like these. Put them together and you do indeed get a "crooked cross." The nuns took it as some sort of a sign, I think. Nuns would appear at my doorway from all over the hospital and point at me with delighted smiles on their faces and say things like, "That's the crooked cross." They all wanted to see me. Even my parents delighted in this. My mother loved to call me the Crooked Cross. My father seemed to stand a little taller when he heard it. It seemed to make everyone happy—even me. I didn't mind the nickname at all. It kind of made me feel special. The significance of my scar wasn't lost on anyone. In very short order, that was my nickname from all, and soon even the doctors and nurses were calling me the Crooked Cross. I think it was great and a fine thing that all those good people at St. Francis hospital who saved my life were able to name the medical miracle that they pulled off. It was good for all of us.

Of course, after however many days it took—again, I don't remember how long it was—it was time to take the stitches out.

As they did after the first operation, they took out the stitches from the secondary wounds first, where I had been connected to the heart-lung machine, my wrists, inner elbows and ankles. Then it was time to remove the stitches from my chest. The bandage was removed, and I was greeted by another huge, hot-pink keloid scar covered with cat-gut stitches. This was the first time I got to see the entire scar, the first time I got to see how my body had again been changed. I had been looking forward to that day, the day they would remove my stitches. I was looking forward to the feelings of having my stitches removed. As it was after the first operation, there was something almost divine about the sensation of stitches being removed. Nowadays, they use sutures that dissolve. By using dissolving stitches, the scars are much smaller, and you don't get the big keloids that the old stitches left. Even so, since they've been using dissolving sutures I feel a little cheated that I can no longer look forward to the sensation one gets when stitches are removed, especially after going through the pain of any kind of procedure that involves an incision. Somehow, it just doesn't seem fair.

23

I was discharged from the hospital on November 20, 1959, 30 days after admission. Oddly, I don't remember anything about that day. I don't remember leaving the hospital, the ride or arriving home. I'm sure I found my bedroom just as sterile, just as lacking in any sign of my presence as I did after the first operation and having the same impact as before. I'm sure the relic of Padre Pio was safety-pinned to my pillow as before, and I'm sure the house felt just as alien to me this time as it did the first. I know that the disconnect between me and my siblings was greater still, but, in all, I don't remember that day.

But I remember other things. For one, I had to take a certain medication called Filobon, an iron rich multivitamin. It consisted of a big, white capsule that had a rubbery feel to it. It didn't appear to have two halves like most capsules but seemed like it was made with one solid coating. You could squeeze this pill in the middle and it would flex. But I hated taking that pill; hated it. My mother would grow impatient with me when it was time for me to take it because I always put up such a fight about it. I told her it tasted bad and my mother would tell me that pills, especially capsules, didn't have a taste. But it did, I would insist, and therefore whenever it was time to take one I would fight my mother.

And it did taste awful.

It wasn't until maybe 30 or 40 years later when my brother, Michael, confessed to my mother and me that they—they being Peter, Michael and Neiani—were dipping the pills in witch hazel. I had mixed feelings on learning that while my mother threw her head back with a big "Ahhhhh," and said, "No wonder you always fought me when it was time to take them." I laughed at the time, but underneath something else was going on. I understood. I didn't like it, but I understood. This was nothing more than another symptom of the resentment that my siblings had towards the special treatment I was getting. I think this fact flew right over my mother's head when Michael confessed. It was unintended, but once I was home from the hospital, a very real "us versus them" mentality had developed between my family and my mother and me.

My siblings were too young to understand the reasons for my mother's overwrought treatment of me, and this dichotomy started at such a young age for them that it became the normal family dynamic, so much so that as they grew older, living with it became more and more the normal family way. All they saw through their young eyes was that I got special treatment from my mother and they didn't, and since this had become the norm, they simply never questioned the why or the wherefore. To them it just was.

What they never understood, however, was that I didn't want to be treated in a special way. They saw the fence my mother had built between us and them, but they always assumed I *wanted* that special treatment, that I wanted to be on my mother's side of the fence. But I didn't. What they could never see was that what was a fence for them was a cage for me, and what kept them out was, for me, the bars of a prison that kept me locked-up behind that fence, that prison with my mother. They never realized in all that time that I was peering out, face between the bars, wishing for my freedom, wishing I was on the other side with them.

I was right that night in the hospital when I waved to them from the ward window and felt that geologic shift beneath my feet, that earthquake whose fault line became a chasm no family member could cross. There was no way for my siblings, and even my parents for that matter, to truly understand what I had been through. No one in the family really saw what had occurred while I was in there. I had been alone for all those procedures and operations. I had been alone when I watched children—children just like me—leave and never come back. I had been alone all those boring days and scary nights. I had been alone for Last Rites and all the other things that happened to me inside those buildings. There was no way I could expect my brothers and sister to understand what had happened to me all those weeks that I had been gone. I knew it then and, unfortunately, it proved to be true. You don't know how many times I've wished that I was wrong that evening, but I wasn't.

Here is more proof of the disconnect, that tectonic shift. From then till now, not one member of my family has ever, *ever* asked me a single question about all that time I spent in the hospital, or what was done to me or how I felt about any of it. Not *any* family member—not ever. And I understand why. It's simple, really. They all thought that they already knew. We certainly know from that incident on Lido Beach that my mother could barely deal with what *she* went through, let alone what is was like for me. And from my siblings' point of view my mother's overindulgence overwhelmed any curiosity they might have had in the first place. Once the resentments started to build, everyone put on their armor; the resentments became their chainmail. Why would they be curious about the very thing they resented? Would you? I doubt it. Would I? I doubt it.

As for me, again, all of this was my fault. I felt powerless at not being able to break through the bonds of my mother's overindulgence. It made me feel weak and helpless. I just knew that if I was only stronger I could stop the bad blood developing inside my family. But because of me, because I'd become sick, because I was too weak to fight off my mother, the family would never be the same again. These two facts always made me smolder with shame and guilt; shame at my weakness and guilt for what I'd done to the family. No one ever knew this was how I felt, and that too was my fault because in my weakness I never found a way to express it. Before too long, I had created a perfect feedback loop of guilt and no one in the family knew it but me.

24

Home life sure was different. When I came home from the hospital I was not healthy enough to go back to my first-grade class. To make sure that I wouldn't fall too far behind my classmates and be left back a grade, my parents brought in a home tutor. I remember her and my home lessons in a vague general sense. I don't remember her name except that there was a "Mrs." before it and that she was a brunette, most likely in her mid-forties and wore her hair in a typical and—even for the day—conservative style. She was a bit portly and both kind and pleasant.

I don't remember her wearing any other color than black; she might have, I just don't remember it. Our kitchen became my classroom and the table became my desk, even though I now can't recount even one lesson I was taught at that table. What I do remember most was that I absolutely hated those home-tutored lessons. I was tired and in no mood for instruction, but, in retrospect, home tutoring was better than being left back a grade. I also remember that when the lesson was over, it wasn't uncommon for my mother and the tutor to speak afterwards for almost as long a time as my lessons were. I got homework, and I did it immediately after the tutor left, making those sessions at the table seem interminable.

I don't remember how my home schooling affected my siblings. I don't know if they were jealous that I got to stay home while they went to school, or if this was something that they understood was a necessity for me. The fact that I don't remember any kind of reactions to it leads me to believe that my home tutoring was a non-event for them.

We didn't live too far from Linder Place Elementary School in Malverne. My brothers always walked to school, as did almost every other kid back then. In those days walking to and from school was the norm and it was something to look forward to. When it was time for me to return to school, however, I was too weak to walk. Since we only had one car and my father used it to drive to 195 Broadway in New York City, (what was then corporate headquarters for AT&T), I had to take a taxi.

Want to know how to get the attention of other children, and not necessarily in the best way? Take a taxi to school; that'll do it. It always embarrassed me whenever I pulled up to the school in a bright yellow taxi and exited, or when school had ended for the day to go into the taxi that was there waiting for me, always on time, always bright yellow. Either way, I couldn't help but notice the stares from my classmates and the other kids in the higher grades. It would have had the same effect if I had gone to school wearing a big sign proclaiming I'M DIFFERENT. My sister was a grade behind me, kindergarten, and she shared the morning taxi with me to school. My brothers had both already moved on to a different school. Fortunately, I only had to take a cab for a few months, and thereafter was able to walk to school on my own. But taking a taxi for as long as I had already done its damage, setting me apart from the other children. I didn't get to hang around and talk to the other kids after school, joke around with them, forge bonds with them. Instead, I went right from the school door, passing the kids who were congregating and goofing around, and right into the waiting taxi.

I had attended school for about a month and a half before I was pulled out to have the second operation and was out longer than I had been in school. School was now just as alien a place for me as my first day in the hospital had been. I'm certain the teacher had spoken to the class about my situation before my return, and I don't remember any of the children being mean to me in the first grade. But it was hard for me to fit in. Think about all that had happened to me in less than two years, about what my actual reality had been. And then, just as suddenly as it had started, I was back in a situation where everything was supposed to be normal where everyone, from my parents on down, expected me to be an ordinary kid living an ordinary life. Just months earlier I was being given Last Rites and then I was supposed to be just another regular kid. But I wasn't. I'd missed some of the most vital time during which children are socialized with one another. I'd seen death up close, and I held a secret, a crooked cross of hot pink keloid scars that branded me as being different from the rest hidden only by my shirt. It was difficult to relate not only with children but adults as well, none of whom had come as close to the reality of their own mortality as had I with mine. In writing this I realize that my father should have been the one to understand; after all, he had fought another man to the death in order to save his own life. But with the way adults thought of children in those days, I don't think he ever made the connection. It's a shame, really, as we both could have been each other's saviors. We had a chance to understand something about each other that no one else in the family could have fathomed and it might have made us especially close as father and son. We could have healed each other and ended the internal nightmares that haunted both of us. Even when we were both adults, neither of us made that connection, made that realization.

Talk about a lost opportunity.

25

As you can imagine, doctors and visits to the doctors were still a huge part of my life, as was St. Francis Hospital. Dr. Balboni had his office at the end of a long, dark, narrow and winding hallway. A little way from his office was a wooden phone booth. I used play in it while my parents spoke to the doctor after my exams. Balboni and my parents were more than likely pleased with my sojourns down this hall as it gave them a chance to speak with one another away from my presence. When I was there, however, they would revert back to the tried and true method of using hushed tones and big words. Didn't matter, I knew what was going on anyway.

My instincts told me that I wasn't out of the woods yet: and I wasn't. Years later, I learned from my mother that no one expected me to live past ten. They never told me or my siblings. I don't think teachers were informed of this information, either. My parents just stuck to their strategy of treating me like a normal child. I'm grateful that they did. It allowed me to continue my own tactic of bullying my heart. But as is true in all things, along with the good came some bad. As time moved me farther and farther from the days of hospitalization, and I had moved out of the first grade, it became more difficult for people to remember what I had been through. I would often wish that if something had to be wrong with me, instead of a heart problem, which stayed hidden in my chest, that I'd had something else, something that was easily apparent, like a limp or anything that would say there was good reason to remember I was fragile. But heart troubles don't show themselves to the outside world in such a demonstrative fashion. To look at me, you wouldn't know that a life-and-death struggle was still going on. I was on the small side, but other kids were shorter. I was the very definition of *skinny*, but other children were thin, too. No, to look at me, there was nothing in my outward appearance that would let you know that I was still a child with a serious heart problem. So, as time went on, bullies found me to be a favorite target, and I became even more withdrawn with every passing day.

I did have a few friends during grade school, but the operative word here was *few*. Gym became a nightmare for me. I was too weak to do anything, and the locker room became a place that put a bull's eye on my back. After just a few sessions of gym class, I complained to my mother and got a doctor's note excusing me from gym. The bullies noticed.

I became aware that I didn't have such a problem with the girls in my class as I did with the boys. It wasn't uncommon for me to have friendships with them. They didn't care that I couldn't throw a ball, (nobody had ever taught me) or that I didn't go to gym class.

But there were a few things I was good at physically. Kickball was my favorite. We used to play it during recess. Nowadays, schools don't allow children to play kickball because if you're hit with the ball and you're called out, it means you lose. Too many of today's generation of parents think this is terrible for their children's self-esteem, that their precious little ones can never be allowed to lose. What hooey. I often was called out. It made me try harder not to be called out in the next game. I was a wiry little thing and for some reason I did pretty well at playing kickball. And contrary to current thinking, it was good for my self-esteem. It showed me and the other kids that there was something physical I could do. I wasn't the best, but I was better than a lot of the other kids. For reasons I didn't understand but was certainly grateful for, the bullies left me alone when we were playing kickball, and never tried to single me out or gang-up on me during a game. No one ever tried to stop me from playing. I was allowed into every game, which I can't say for almost any other physical activity at school. When playing kickball, for that brief time at least, I really was just one of the kids. I'm grateful they hadn't banned kickball when I was a child. The fact that it is banned today makes me feel sorry for today's kids.

26

At this time of my life, the bullying directed my way usually took the form of being excluded from the main group of kids and relentless taunting. But a couple of incidents really stand out in my mind. The first incident involved the tallest kid in the class. I won't name him, but in addition to being tallest, he was also the class smart-aleck. If someone was either going to talk back to the teacher or have a wisecrack answer to a question a teacher asked, it would be him.

One day during recess he started to make fun of my thumbs. I don't remember the actual words, but I do remember how much they hurt. Okay, it was my lot that I'd be the most unpopular kid in the class. I got it. I read the memo. I could almost deal with that. All those months I'd spent alone in both the hospital and my bed at home had made it possible for me to turn inward during taunting sessions. Of course, I hated it and wished it was different, but it wasn't and wouldn't be, so I just dealt with it the best as I could. I was always being teased and made fun of; as a result, I became introverted and built a wall for the hurtful words to bounce off. But when he started to make fun of my thumbs in front of a laughing gaggle of my classmates, those words were as sharp as any scalpel I'd been under in the hospital. Those taunts about my thumbs cut through my protective wall as easily as if it was built of wet tissue paper. I could take the taunting, the being made fun of. I could take the occasional bully pushing me to the ground inside a laughing circle of cruel cowards. But I couldn't take that. For some reason, that was the line for me that couldn't be crossed. I took the only action I could think to take; I went to the teacher and told her what he had been saying.

My teachers knew I was the runt of the class. I knew it bothered them, some more than others. I had always thought of this teacher as belonging to the latter camp. But when I told her about him making fun of my thumbs, I was surprised to see that this bit of information really upset her.

I stood outside the doorway of our classroom as she spoke to him about it. I remember hearing her say, "How would you feel if it was you who had thumbs like that and people made fun of you?" She didn't know I was there and that I had overheard her comment. But even that comment, said in my defense, hurt. I don't remember anything else she said, but whatever it was, she stopped it. Neither he nor any other kid ever made fun of my thumbs again. This held true as I moved from school to school and town to town. I think that somehow by standing up for myself in that instance, it did something to me, changed something inside me that somehow others could see: my thumbs became the line you couldn't cross. But my "telling" on him had its own effect on me. I had never tattled to a teacher before about the way I was being treated and never did again after that. It made me feel weak and helpless to have done so, even if it was just this once. So, on the one hand I was pleased that I had stopped my thumbs from being objects of derision, but on the other hand, to my mind, I had shamed myself. To this day, whenever I think of this event, I still think of that internal conflict and still feel the shame. Funny how these things can last, isn't it?

The next incident happened in fourth grade, my last year at Linder Place. It was Valentine's Day. I had spent the previous night writing Valentine cards. I had one for each kid. My mother had insisted I do it this way because, "we didn't want to leave anyone out and hurt their feelings," she had said to me. I went to school that day excited to see how many cards I would get. I knew that if I got any cards it would most likely be from those who had done what I did—made a card for each classmate. But that didn't matter to me. I was full of anticipation for how my cards would be received and, mostly, to see how many cards I would get. I really didn't expect too many. When it came time to pass out the cards, they were all put in a big box and the teacher would reach in, pull a card out and call the name of the intended recipient out loud to the class and then deliver the card to the addressee.

In the beginning of this exercise it was no surprise to me that my name hadn't been called. Of course, the "popular kids" got the most cards. I expected that. But soon, every one of my class-mates had been called, some several times, and still, my name hadn't been called. Every time a popular kid got a card it was accompanied by sounds of approval from all of the others. I noticed when someone got one of my cards the reaction from the recipient and the rest of the class was, well, tepid at best.

Finally, my name was called. The card was from a girl who had done what I did: made a card for everyone in the class. This girl didn't particularly like me. She treated me like most of my classmates did, and normally wouldn't give me the time of day.

She was never mean to me outright, but always acted as if I didn't exist. So, that was it. Just one card for me, the only kid in the class to get only one Valentine card. And, of course, the whole class knew that I'd only received the one. I really should have expected it, but I didn't. Out of a class of 30-something kids, I just assumed I would get five cards, maybe ten, even if only because, like me, they had made one for everybody. I guess I had a little fantasy going in my head, a little dream that I wasn't as disliked as my everyday school life indicated; a little wish that somehow things weren't really as bad as they seemed. But I only got the one, and the message it delivered to me from the rest of the class was as clear as a bell. Now there was no doubt in anyone's mind—not mine, not all the kids, not the teacher's—what their regard for me was, and my stupid little fantasies be damned.

I went home that day completely and utterly humiliated. I couldn't even bring myself to tell my mother or the rest of the family what had happened that day. Why spread my humiliation? Why give my brothers more fodder to use against me? Why give my father even more reason to be disappointed with me? Why give my mother additional reasons to strengthen the walls she built dividing her and me from the rest of the family? No, this one I had to keep to myself.

It was almost impossible for me to drag myself back to school the next day.

27

My father was a remarkable man. Born into poverty in the Bronx, New York, he shared the same bed with his four brothers. His father died while he was a boy. He was a street kid, but not a thug. He was raised correctly. He always wanted to do what was right, and, in particular, what was right for him. He had ambition and drive. He put himself through school and played college football. He studied art and got his degree. Now all of that would be pretty impressive accomplishments for anyone, but one of my father's achievements stands out with me the most. It was how he taught himself to play piano.

Learning how to play the piano was my father's burning desire from a young age. The fact that he was poor and didn't even have access to a piano, let alone the money for lessons, wasn't going to stop him. So, he got an idea and acted on it. He found a long piece of cardboard and traced out a piano keyboard on it, life size, and then correctly colored the appropriate "keys" black or white. He then somehow obtained piano exercise books and started to learn how to play the scales, while using the correct fingering. He would practice like this for hours a day and for days that turned into years. When he was finally able to gain access to a real piano, he already knew how to play it. He did this without ever hearing a note that he played from his cardboard cutout, but by hearing the notes clearly in his mind.

By the time I came around, our home in Malverne already had a baby grand in the living room. This was my parents' second home and I have no idea if this piano was in that house too or if it was new to this one. I never gave that a thought. What mattered was that the piano was there at all. My father would play on weekend mornings and I would go under the piano and sit there and listen. This was my safe haven. Under there, covered by the magical blanket of my father's music, I could relax; I was safe from the rest of the family. My brothers couldn't taunt me, and my mother couldn't smother me. No, here I was safe and, more importantly, I could be close to my father, too. We never spoke about it, but I think he liked the idea that I was drawn to his music. And, he was good, too. Rich in chords, mostly played in the middle registers, show tunes, 40's and 50's classics and jazz seemed to come out of my father's fingertips like magic. His music would transport me to a wonderful world of melody, a different world that could only be gained on those weekends with me sitting under the soundboard of that baby grand, where just above that, little felt-tipped hammers struck the strings of the piano's harp, as my father's fingers effortlessly flew over the keyboard. Not only did I feel safe there, but I learned to love music there, too.

I learned to love music from both of my parents. We had a high-end stereo and when my father wasn't playing the piano that stereo would fill the entire house with everything from opera to jazz, Sinatra to Italian music. My mother sang as well as Ella did, no kidding, and had a shot at becoming a professional singer when she was younger. But her hopes were dashed when her cruel mother told her if she did that, she'd be a whore. Old Italians were funny like that. My mother should have pursued her dreams because to that kind of an Italian she became a whore anyway the day she got her nursing degree. It was all connected to the idea that those professions were filled by "loose women." But it was my father's piano that so effectively reached a spot deep inside of me. Jazz piano still transports me, still makes my soul fly, still has a calming effect on me. But not like it did when I was sitting under Daddy's piano in Malverne.

There are two things I'd give almost anything for: to taste my mother's lasagna again and to sit under that piano while my father played. For the chance to do both at once, I'd give up everything I have in this world.

28

That's pretty much how my life in Malverne went: bullies to contend with at school, the taunting from my brothers at home, the suffocating affections of my mother, the disappointment of my father, and the alienation that my mother's over-attention caused between me and the rest of the family. My siblings never really understood that I had nowhere else to go. I wasn't any good at sports. I was never taught how to throw a ball, not by my father, nor for that matter not by any of my gym teachers, either. Look, I was the youngest brother, and I know that all younger brothers get taunted to some degree or another. Was I taunted more than most? I really don't know. I don't have a frame of reference to judge by. I do know, however, that it probably seemed worse to me because it seemed like I never caught a break: Bullies at school, my brothers at home. Most likely they weren't any worse than any other older brothers were to their youngest siblings. I just wanted a break.

There was a group of children who lived on my block and I got along with them pretty well. We would get together and play war, running around our yards with plastic machine guns, taking turns at who were the Americans and who were the Germans. All of us had fathers who had served in World War II and we were all proud of them. And I had my bike. I loved my bike. In those days a child could just get on a bicycle and disappear for the whole day, as long as you were home in time for supper. No cell phones, no knee, elbow pads or helmets.

Remarkably, none of us were ever taken by a stranger or killed for want of safety gear. I used to travel all around town on my bike, always stopping to explore a new field or part of town I wasn't familiar with. I loved to explore, and because I was alone much of the time, I spent a great deal of my time just riding around exploring the neighborhood.

Michael, it turns out, was the one who taught me to ride a bicycle. One beautiful spring or summer day, I can't remember which it was, we took the training wheels off my bike and walked it over to the empty lot across from the library, right across the street from my school. Michael picked that lot because it was all grass, well groomed with no stones or other kinds of debris to get hurt on if, well, really, *when* I fell. It had a smooth, even surface except for a large depression almost center. He steadied me on the bike, one hand holding a handle bar, the other the back of the seat, and when we were both reasonably sure I was holding steady, he would launch me with a push on the back of my seat.

Of course, I fell a bunch of times; after all, that was what we both expected. But it was all so much fun, especially when I started to get the feeling that I was beginning to learn how to balance. And then, of course, I did learn. Michael was as triumphant about my accomplishment as I was, and I rode the bike home while he walked beside me. I loved being his little brother that day; I think as much as he loved being my big brother.

There was one other day I spent with Michael that I remember as one of the best days of my entire life. We left the house to walk into town and, while I really don't remember what it was that we did exactly, I remember us laughing for most of the time. The event that I do remember from that day I will never forget.

The Long Island Railroad train tracks ran right through the center of town. Naturally there were gates that came down to stop both cars and pedestrians. We were walking back home and had just crossed the tracks and there in the sidewalk right in front of us was a big crack in the cement. Without saying a word to each other we both jumped up and landed smack across that crack. At the exact moment that our feet touched the ground the warning bell for the track gates started to ring. To us it was magic and, somehow, we both knew that because our feet hit the crack at the exact same time, was the *real* reason why that bell went off when it did. We had such a great time that day. But the dynamics roiling inside our home made sure that those kinds of days would be the exception and not the rule. What a pity.

29

A t this stage of life, my biggest concern was bullies. No matter where I seemed to go, no matter what I did, I attracted bullies. Even in a hospital.

A few years after my last heart operation, I was having a real problem with strep throat. Several times a year I was having serious bouts of it. This went on for a few years. Once again, it alerted my mother's momma bear instincts. She thought the problem was my tonsils, as did my doctors, and once again she went to war with the doctors to have them removed. I'm not sure what the reluctance was on the part of the doctors to not remove my tonsils, but my mother was insistent. And finally, I was admitted to St. Luke's Hospital in New York City to have my tonsils removed. There was no doubt that my mother thought that my getting seriously ill several times a year outweighed any of the cardiac concerns that my doctors had.

So off to the city I went for yet another operation. I remember that this hospital had a very different feel than that of St. Francis. It wasn't just that this one was in the city, whereas St.

Francis was in the suburbs, but in this hospital there were no nuns and no large crosses decorating the rooms. No doctor, no nurse mistook the seriousness of the surgery I was about to have. After all, not only was I medical history, but I was still a very frail patient. I don't remember the name of the doctor who was going to perform the surgery, but I can still see him very clearly in my mind. He was kind and had a face that always seemed to be adorned with a smile. Like most children who were to get a tonsillectomy, I was looking forward to the promise of all the ice cream I could eat in the recovery phase. When I think about it, this doctor treated me like an equal, not a little kid. It was almost as if we had become partners in crime. I had heard stories of children who had tonsillectomies and got to take their tonsils home. I wanted to take mine home, too. I remember being in my hospital bed with this doctor and my parents standing beside it when I asked the doctor if I could have my tonsils. I remember my mother's reaction quite clearly, her face a combination of horror and defiance. I also remember the doctor's face. His reaction to my mother's reaction was a combination of humor and mischief. His eyes told me that I would be going home with my tonsils in a jar. I don't think my mother was very happy about this, but the doctor's mischievous grin set me at ease and told me not to worry about it. And I didn't.

That night, the night before the operation, the nurses had taken me to a common playroom for children. At first, I was the only child in the room. I had found a little toy truck and was playing with it at the far end of the room. Soon several other boys entered and started playing at the opposite end. Used to being by myself, I didn't even try to engage the boys and just continued to play with my little toy truck. But out of the corner of my eye I could see that I had started to become the focus of the other boys' attention. I started to get that feeling in my gut that I always got when I knew that soon I was going to become the new toy for these boys to play with.

It's always the same with bullies. The largest boy is the ringleader, followed by a couple of smaller boys. My impression of bullies is the same now as it was then; they are all cowards, regardless of their age or circumstance. Sure enough, the group of three approached me with the largest boy at point. I was still down on the ground playing with my truck. As they approached, I kind of went into a zone, not quite my cave nor up with my seagull, but a place where a large part of me just shut down and accepted the inevitable. And the inevitable did come. I don't remember what was said or what the taunts were, but I was obviously being made fun of and the object of their derision. I was easily the smallest among them, and, of course, that is what attracts the bullies in the first place, cowards that they are.

The encounter, fortunately, was brief. I offered no resistance of any kind and did not answer any of their taunts. I had learned one thing when it came to bullies, and that was to offer as little entertainment value for them as possible so they would get bored and move on to something else. I wouldn't look any of them in the eye, and I didn't make a sound. And while that strategy worked in keeping this encounter brief, it still didn't end until the largest boy had kicked the truck out of my hand and took it from me. With my truck as the trophy for their bravery, the bully and his entourage left triumphant. And while they left me alone for the rest of my time in that room, it left me wondering what was it about me that everybody seemed to hate? What was it about me that was so bad that no matter where I went, my home, my school or even a hospital, I just could not get away without being bullied in one way or another? It wasn't just that this bully took a truck from me; that day, that bully took something from me that would trouble me for many years to come.

Call it my pride, my self-worth, whatever you want to call it, I lost a hunk of it that day.

I often wonder about that boy, that particular bully. What kind of a man did he finally become? Is he still a bully? Is he still a sniveling coward? Does he beat his wife and children? Does he kick the dog when he comes home? Is he helping to raise another generation of bullies as his father did? Is he still the weak, pathetic, insecure little bully that he was then? Who knows? I would be lying to you if I didn't admit that I've fantasized that one day he tried to bully the wrong person. Someone who, to his great surprise, was able to strongly, and without doubt, put him in his place and teach him a well-deserved lesson. One can only hope.

Despite this latest encounter with a bully, the tonsillectomy went well, I no longer got strep throat and I did go home with my tonsils in a jar, much to my delight and my mother's horror and dismay. Thanks, doc!

30

My brothers used to go to a sleep-away camp located on the North Shore of Long Island called Camp Alvernia. Both of my brothers were terrific athletes and they always came home bearing trophies and awards they had won at camp. When my mother told me I would be going too, I knew instinctively that this was a bad idea. I knew everyone at camp would be expecting another Taibbi athlete, another kid who would be popular. In my experience from school, I knew such expectations would never bode well for me. I knew it would be a set-up for disaster. And, of course, it was.

Almost right away I could see that same kind of disappointment in the eyes of the counselors that I had often seen in the eyes of teachers who had my brothers in their classes before me. As soon as I would see that look I would feel the shame rising within me. But at least none of them would bully me. But on the other hand, none of them would really go out of their way to protect me either. In the very early sixties, men were supposed to be men, and, in some strange and bizarre way, I think that the counselors thought that the mistreatment of me by the other campers would somehow be good for me.

It wasn't long before I caught the attention of another bully and his entourage. What fun it was for them to be able to pick on the little sick kid to prove how manly they were. And so it transpired that on one sunny afternoon I had my first encounter with them. There was a recreation hall opposite my cabin, and the space between it and my cabin was used as an assembly area in the mornings. Right in the middle of this space was where this encounter and all subsequent other encounters with these four boys took place. As I said before, bullies never act alone. As usual, the leader was bigger than the other three boys who followed him. I still have a fair recollection of what he looked like. He was more than a good head taller than me and taller than the other boys, as well. His hair was sandy-color and he was slightly pudgy. His build suggested that one day he would be on a high school football team. The four of them walked up to me, calling me names and laughing. At first I just stood in front of them as I absorbed the name-calling and ridicule. After a few moments of this, name-calling wasn't enough, and Pudgy started to shove me backwards by pushing me with both of his hands against my shoulders. Every time he pushed I was forced to take a step or two back. What I hadn't noticed was that one of the boys had slipped behind me and gotten down on his hands and knees. One or two shoves later, I fell backwards against him and fell on my back. That brought pure, hysterical enjoyment to the four of them; they were literally bending over and slapping their knees with laughter.

When I got up, Pudgy grabbed me, stuck out his leg, and threw me back down to the ground with some sort of karate move. More hysterical laughter. But I got up again and, once again, he easily threw me over his leg back onto the ground—hard. More hysterical laughter. Every time I got up, he did the same thing. I had no way of defending myself from this, but I refused to be thrown to the ground, so I kept getting up. He must've thrown me five or six times, not including the original backwards trip. Finally, I got the hint and stayed on the ground with the four boys standing above me laughing as hard as they could.

This became a daily routine. Every single day I would be set upon by these four thugs. Every single day I would get thrown to the ground five to seven times. How the counselors never saw this happening, I still don't understand, since this was taking place in the very center of the camp. This was the only group of bullies I encountered at this camp, but it was enough to make my time there miserable. They never attacked me anywhere else, but it made me fearful that anywhere I went at any time they could attack me and throw me to the ground. I started writing my parents every day to take me home. I begged them to come and get me. I was supposed to be at this camp for a month, but my pleading letters to my parents finally worked and I came home after about two weeks.

Home was strange now, because my brothers and sister were still at camp. I think my parents had wanted this time to be for themselves, but, of course, I had to ruin it for them. This was the first time I was alone in that house without the other children. It felt strange and empty and yet I loved it. Our part-time maid, Evelyn, who was African-American and who I dearly loved, was a great comfort to me during this time. I think Evelyn had a handle on the dynamics of our family. After all, she was a part of the family, which is what we all considered her, and as a part of our family it was natural for her to have this understanding. I spent most of my time happily in my room building models of rockets and Evelyn would come in and look at what I was building with genuine interest. It's funny how when I think of this time, I almost always think of Evelyn.

I told my parents I would never go back to that camp, and I never did.

31

And while it's true that I never did go back to that camp, I did, however, go to another camp the next year. Camp Molloy was a Catholic boys' camp out in Mattituck, Long Island and situated on the shore of Lake Laurel. My parents seemed to think that camp would be good for me, therefore I was going to go. I think this was part of their plan to make me have as normal a childhood as possible. Of course, *normal* meant that we never spoke about anything that happened to me in the hospital or of my conditions. I think in the minds of my parents, they took the notion of "out of sight, out of mind" a step beyond; thus, I found myself at another camp that next June.

Like the last camp, the scenery was beautiful. And like the last camp there was a bully and his entourage of thugs who thought I would make a wonderful plaything for their amusement. But this camp was different from the rest in that I had started to learn how to make friends. I had met several other boys who I hung out and shared camp activities with. I got along very well with these boys and looked forward to seeing them every day. I certainly would not include us as part of the athletic crowd, as it was our lack of athleticism that was pretty much the glue that held us together. What I had yet to realize was that I was quite strong, and I would find out just how strong not more than a few days after becoming this other bully's favorite toy.

It's like a scene from a bad movie. You know, the kind of movies that all seem to have the same plot, the same type of characters, all playing out in the same type of storyline. Like the last bully, this one was at least a head taller and several years older than me. His little sycophant gang, this time numbering four, did as all the other bully hangers-on did. They looked up to him and would do whatever he said. Our first confrontation was in an open field on a beautiful summer's day. Like a bad Western, they approached me deliberately and with malice of intent. You didn't need my background in bullies to see a mile away that they meant me no good.

And, just as in the last camp, the ringleader had sandy-colored hair, but he was thin. He had the build of a track-and-field star. And like the same disgusting script that seemed to keep repeating itself in a continuous, sickening loop in my life, they just walked up to me, their taunts starting even before they reached me. I don't really remember how it happened, as I had gone into a zone preparing myself for the worst. What I do remember is that I suddenly found myself on the ground, on my back, surrounded by a laughing bunch of goons.

This happened again on the next day, and the day after that. But something happened on the fourth day that took me, and them, quite by surprise.

We were again in the same field at the same spot. I imagine

there was something about the location that gave them courage. Maybe it was because we were out of sight from the counselors or maybe it was something else that made them feel safe. But on this fourth day, I again found myself on the ground, my back hurting, my ears filled with their ridicule and laughter. Then something in me snapped. And, I do mean *snapped*. Suddenly my vision went dark until just a thin tunnel of light was visible. I felt a huge and violent rage exploding somewhere deep inside. I had never experienced anything like it before, but I found that it overtook me. I just went where it led; it was as if I didn't have any choice in the matter. By this time, I'd gotten onto my hands and knees and all I could see was a tall, sandy-haired bastard who I wanted to destroy. They were so busy laughing they didn't notice the change in my body language or the rage in my eyes and face. I sprang up onto my feet as fast as a cat and ran after the kid with everything I had. I will always remember the look of shock in his eyes when he realized I was coming for him. By the time he did, I was almost upon him and he didn't have time to react. I didn't know how to fight; after all, no one ever taught me how to throw a ball so certainly no one ever taught me how to defend myself, either. But my rage would be my instructor.

Just before I reached him, I tucked my head down and I rammed him with my shoulder into his right-side rib cage with all my might. He went flying backwards with me hanging onto him for dear life. He landed on his back hard, hard enough it might've even knocked some of the wind out of him. I'm not sure, but it didn't matter because now he was mine. Before either of us knew it, I was sitting on his chest, my knees holding down his arms, and I started to pummel his face. Like I said, I didn't know how to fight, so I certainly didn't know how to punch. But what I was doing to him was just as good. I had turned my fists into hammers, my arms pivoting up and down at my elbows like some machine from the industrial age gone mad. Up and down, up and down my fists went, every one of them landing directly on his face. I was hitting his nose, his mouth, his eyes and his cheeks. I really wasn't aiming at any particular target, but every blow landed. I was literally pounding his face with my fists. His entourage stood back, mouths agape, shock registering on their faces. The screams I was hearing were coming from the bully pinned beneath me; the blood from his nose was on my fists.

Screaming. Maybe that was the factor that made me such an easy target. I never screamed. I never went to a counselor after an attack. I always just took it and took it. But not with this big, brave bully. No, not him. He was screaming like a little girl in a short pink dress. I don't know why, but there was something about his screams and yells that only made me hit him harder. I couldn't tell you how long this went on for, but it only ended when *two* counselors had to peel me off him. All I do know is that every punch I delivered represented each encounter I ever had with all the other bullies in my life. I was finally striking back blow for blow what bullies had been doing to me for years.

Not only was the bully in shock along with his entourage, but the counselors were, too. I know one of the counselors was reprimanding me, but I didn't hear one word of it. They never reprimanded him after he beat me, so *screw them*, I thought. I didn't care what they were saying to me. And besides, I was too busy enjoying the moment and the discovery that bullies could be beaten. Before that incident the idea that I could beat a bully had never even occurred to me. In my mind it was just my lot that I would be the subject of bullying, the way it was my lot that I had to spend so much time in hospitals.

Something inside of me changed that afternoon. I wasn't sure what it was, but for that moment all I wanted to do was enjoy the feeling of sheer exhilaration. For the first time in my life I had won something. I didn't get a trophy or a patch to wear on my jacket, but I can still see that kid's bloody face under the hammers of my fists. That was my trophy. That was my prize, and I'd won it fair and square.

The next day I saw the bully with his little group pretty much in the same place. Do you know what I did? I rammed him again, knocked him on his back, pinned him with my knees and started to hammer his face once again. I did it for the pure enjoyment of it. I did it simply because I wanted to. *I did it because I wanted to bully him. How do **you** like it, you little piece of shit?*

If there was ever a question that bullies are just cowards, one only has to look at his entourage. There were four of them. I was easily outnumbered, but not one of them tried to help their friend. It was obvious they were afraid of me and I took a great deal of satisfaction in knowing that. Once again, I didn't stop until I was removed by counselors. One of the counselors seemed to know that I had been bullied by this kid, but he wasn't happy that I was returning the favor. Once again, I was admonished. Once again, I didn't hear it. The satisfaction just felt too good. So, what do you think happened the day after that? You guessed it: I did it again. And I did it again the day after that. The counselors probably think that I stopped bullying him because they told me I had to stop. But that wasn't the reason. I stopped because after the last time I set upon this kid, and the counselors had again separated us, I overheard one say to the other as they were walking away, "That one is a bully." He was referring to me. I never felt so proud.

From there on in I never went after him again. I didn't need to; he was afraid of me, as was his little group of thugs. After all, it was the counselors who had branded *me* the bully. Whenever he saw me he would shy away; *they* would shy away. That was good enough for me. Now, for the first time of my camp life, I could enjoy the experience without having to be in fear I would be set-upon at any moment. Word had gotten around with the other kids and suddenly I was more popular. My circle of friends expanded, and I noticed that the other "tough guys" at the camp gave me a wide berth. For the first time, I was having a great time at camp—until I got sick.

It had started with a cough, but by the time I took myself to the infirmary I was quite ill. The camp nurse wasn't sure, but she thought I might have pneumonia. Of course, they knew my medical history and this finding prompted an emergency call to my parents. My father came to the camp and picked me up in his black 1960 Cadillac. I was put in the back seat of the car and my father headed straight for St. Francis hospital.

Both of my parents were excellent drivers, my father being the better of the two. I looked on from the back seat and watched my father as he expertly weaved through Long Island daytime traffic. I looked at the speedometer, fascinated by the speedometer's needle as it swung from 80 to 110. All the while, my father's demeanor was that of a man just out for a drive. No motion on the wheel was abrupt; all movements were smooth and precise. I had no fear while we drove at breakneck speed to get to the hospital. My father was hoping that he would get caught for speeding and thereby gain a police escort. But amazingly, that never happened, and we got to the hospital all on our own, all in one piece.

Once there, I was diagnosed not with pneumonia but with pleurisy, an inflammation of the lining of the lung that is worse than pneumonia. I would be spending the rest of what would have been my summer camp time in the hospital. But all was not lost. I had taken down the bully, been tagged a bully by the counselors, and had learned a great lesson. More than that, I took the bully down all by myself. I didn't need a gang to back me up like all the bullies of my past had done. I was better than a bully. I was the avenger for all those who had been bullied. I was the avenger of *my* bullies. It was all okay with me. I was happy. This had been a good summer.

32

At the end of sixth grade, my parents decided it was time to leave Malverne. We moved to an area on the North Shore of Long Island called Brookville. My father had done well for himself and we made the move up. Even today, Brookville is one of the nicest places on Long Island, and not far from Oyster Bay with its beautiful beaches, lovely harbor and access to Long Island sound.

My new school was the Brookville Elementary School, a short walk from my home. Our new home—and it was brand-new—sat on three beautiful acres with well over half an acre of front lawn and woods that got thicker as you went back through the property. It was rural; there were no sidewalks or streetlights, and I thought it was just perfect. I started my new school in the fifth grade and all my classmates had homes at least the equal of mine and many had homes that were much grander. The truth of the matter was that most of my classmates came from families with "established money," or "old money," whereas we were *nouveau riche*, or new money. Those kids and their families had

had money all their lives. I think we stuck out in the neighborhood like a sore thumb. To say that a lot of my classmates were snobs would be to put it mildly. Not all of them, of course, but enough to make us feel the difference. In this regard, the girls were much worse than the boys. We've all had heard that expression of someone having their "nose in the air." I can think of one girl in particular who that expression seemed to be invented for. At every opportunity this brat would let me know that she felt I was inferior to her. Some of the boys were that way too, but with them they manifested it as not belonging in their club. They let you know that at every opportunity; not much in words, but in exclusion and derision. If I thought I'd had it bad in Malverne, what I experienced at the Brookville school made me long for the days of Linder Place. At least in Malverne there was no class distinctions. I found my new male classmates to have a degree of meanness and cruelty that only comes with privilege.

33

So, it's the next summer and once again I'm off to camp and, once again, I'm off to a different camp. This time a Boy Scout camp. I couldn't tell you where it was exactly, but like the others, it was somewhere on Long Island. I think it was further out east, but I can't be sure. The campgrounds were beautiful with lush woodlands that sat next to a body of water. I don't remember if the water was Long Island Sound or a protected bay on either the North or South Shore, but I guess it really doesn't matter, except to say that it was a beautiful location. I took the fact that this was a new camp, with new kids who didn't know me, as an opportunity to learn how to get along with others without being bullied.

Since this was a Boy Scout camp our sleeping quarters were tents on raised wooden platforms that were situated in the thinner part of the woods. I loved it. I can't recall if this was the first time I ever slept out in a tent, and I don't think it was, but I'm sure it was *this* camping experience that made me fall in love with the idea of camping that I still have today. I remember that my bunkmate and I got along quite well. That fact alone made me feel like I was at least gaining some ground in my social skills. I have some good memories from that time at summer camp and none of them included any bullying incidences at all.

I remember one morning, very early just after dawn, waking up in my cot only to find a chipmunk sitting on the floor just inches below my head where I lay. I don't think that I ever had a wild animal that close to me before. I was captivated by him. He was beautiful. I made sure not to move a muscle. I only opened my eyes partly as not to scare him off. He just sat there happily chewing away at something, something he probably found in our tent. Of course, I've seen a chipmunk before, but never so close. That was my first discovery at this camp.

It was also where I discovered cursing.

I couldn't for the life of me tell you how it started, or exactly when, but I knew I needed a strategy to keep the bullies away. Bear in mind that this was the early Sixties, and things were much different than they are today. Cursing was frowned on by all, and I think I thought that if I cursed, it would put the others a little bit off balance when it came to me. It worked. The bigger kids and the bullies didn't know quite what to make of me and my cursing. It somehow put me off limits as someone they could bully and get away with it. It reminds me of a story a friend told me years later.

He was a casual friend, more the friend of my best friend, and he had gone to prison for possession of pot. Let's call him "Paul" to make it easy. Paul told us the story of something he saw while on the lunch line in jail. A new guy had just joined the ranks of the prison population; what the others would call a "fish." According to Paul, he was a little guy, and little guys don't do well in prison. It seems this guy understood that fact and decided to do something about it. He picked the biggest guy in line and just simply attacked him from behind. Screaming and yelling like a mad man, he jumped on his back, and while holding on for dear life, he bit one of the ears of the bigger guy clean off. Paul told us that from then on, no one would go near him because they thought he was crazy and they were afraid of him.

I imagine that my cursing was somewhat analogous to biting someone's ear off. They didn't know what to make of me and were a little leery of me. If I was willing to curse the way I did, what would I do if they tried to do something to me? They wanted to bully me, they just weren't sure it was the smart thing to do, so they left me alone. I distinctly remember one kid in particular. He was both bigger and older than me, and he had his little entourage of hangers-on. It was obvious to me he would have liked to have bullied me, but my profanity put a wall between us that he felt better not to scale. I found it fascinating to watch his reactions towards me. I can still see his dumbfounded face one day on a trail in the woods, a perfect place to attack me. I could see the gears turning in his head as he decided what it was he was going to do. Finally, he called me a name and left with his sycophantic troupe, clearly frustrated by the dilemma I had given him. I had used their cowardice against them and my reward was the first camp experience where I didn't have to keep looking over my shoulder for the next attack. I remember feeling quite triumphant that day. Don't get me wrong, most of the kids still didn't like me, but I had my friends, and all was fine with me.

I learned something else that summer: I was much stronger than I thought. I realized this when our councilors took a large group of us for canoe races.

We'd race in pairs, one canoe against the other until it came down to the last two finalists. I was one of the two finalists.

Oddly, this didn't surprise me. I was good with a canoe; knew how to paddle correctly and really enjoyed canoeing. The boy I was racing in the finals was bigger than me (most of them were) and stronger. But I somehow knew in my gut that I'd win. And I did—by a comfortable margin—to the surprise of the councilors and the other kids. It was kind of like the geeks against the jocks and this geek beat the jock. It made me a pariah with the jocks but a bit of a hero with the geeks. I had beaten everyone involved in that race, and I have to tell you, it felt wonderful. It still does.

Summer at this camp had been great, and I'd finally figured out a strategy to keep the bullies at bay.

34

ummer camp experiences aside, I was still returning to the Brookville school, where my lowly status had firmly been established. My place on the social totem pole would not change and the bullies I had to contend with wouldn't change either. What was different, however, was the form of bullying. Unlike in my previous school or at the summer camps where bullies used physical force, as well as name-calling and exclusion, here at this school nothing physical was ever done to me. But the name-calling and the exclusion were even greater here. I did not have a single friend among my classmates and spent most of my time at school alone.

Phys Ed didn't help. I had a gym teacher, like all the other gym teachers I'd already encountered, who believed all I needed was more physical exercise. But I still wasn't up to it as well as the other students. By this time in my life, around sixth grade, I was still often sickly. I was anemic for a couple of years and didn't have the stamina required, nor the knowledge and skills necessary, to be active in sports.

When it came to gym class baseball games, the teacher would assign two team captains, one of whom was my worst nemesis, and they would get to pick who would be on their team. I was never picked. This one was understandable in the sense that I was the worst player in the class, so having me on a team would be a distinct advantage for the opposing team. One of my most painful memories of this time was when the two team captains got into an actual brawl over which team I would go to. The loser got me.

I wasn't much help to my cause, either. I remember one game when I was out in the field. I really didn't know what I was supposed to do. I was daydreaming, not paying attention, when the ball that was hit was coming right for me. It should have been an easy catch, even for me, but it just went right by me. What should have been an easy out became a home run because of me. That one was absolutely my fault, and everybody involved from all the players on my team to the gym teacher let me know it.

Then there was a school athletic event where our entire class had to participate. It was a track-and-field event. I think it was a race that I lost, but for some reason I was going to get some kind of award, a patch, I think, just because I had participated. Standing in line to receive my prize from the principal, who had set up a little table on the field, I was proud I was finally going to receive something for sports, even if it was for last place. Unfortunately, it was not to happen.

Standing in line in front of me was one of my tormenters, and he had lots to say about my last-place finish. I answered back, and it got a little heated, mostly on his side. The principal looked up from her table and warned us to be quiet. He persisted in his pestering. I said something back, and the principal threw us both out of line. Neither of us would get any prize. What a huge disappointment that was for me, then and even now. That would have been the only thing I would ever have won for doing something athletic in my entire life, and at the last moment it was taken from me. To this day I feel like the principal should have had a better handle on the situation since she knew my position in the school, and I still believe she should have known I wasn't the instigator. But it didn't matter, I was to be denied my prize, to the great satisfaction of that kid who had been tormenting me.

I finally got my mother to produce a note from a doctor saying that I could no longer participate in gym class, but really it was too little, too late.

When I said I didn't have a single friend among my classmates, I wasn't exaggerating. During recess when all the other children would be playing on the field, I was alone. Having no one to play with I took to walking around the field for the recess period. I would walk around the entire perimeter of the field all by myself. The school field was surrounded on three sides by woods, and I would walk around this edge, often exploring and looking for something nature would supply—a new plant, insects, whatever, or just get lost in my own thoughts. Of course, every kid in school and all the teachers would see me do this, but I was getting to a point where I just didn't care anymore. I'm sure it cemented in place whatever they all thought of me already, but being alone also meant for that hour I didn't have to listen to any taunts, and the fact that I was walking out there alone, well, that at least, was *my* choice.

35

Summer was approaching and so was summer camp. But once again, I was going to a different camp. This one as different a summer camp as there could be. It was also the place where I would finally re-invent myself, but that wouldn't occur this particular summer.

It was, I was told by my parents, a camp for children who'd had open-heart surgery. As a matter of fact, that was the price of admission; to be a camper there, one had to have the scars of open-heart surgery. That must have been the attraction for my parents. I would finally be surrounded by children who had much the same experiences that I'd had. I'm sure my parents felt I wouldn't be bullied there and finally be somewhere I would be accepted.

I didn't want to go. I wanted to go back to the Boy Scout camp. But my parents thought this would be better for me. So, my sixth-grade summer was to be partially spent at Madden Farm, in Great Barrington, MA.

Edward J. Madden had been one of the first open-heart

patients. In 1960, he and his wife, Leone, decided to open their summer home in the foothills of the beautiful Berkshire Mountains. It had 300 acres, a stream running through it, was co-ed and only accommodated a small group of us at a time. I would guess the camp population was somewhere around 30 campers.

The property consisted of the main house, a large white farmhouse with a dining area that at one time must have been a huge screened-in porch that had been transformed into the place where the entire camp population, including councilors and the Maddens ate, and several out buildings. One, which looked like it had been a barn at one time, was the rec hall. The lower level of the barn was still a barn where the maintenance equipment for the grounds were kept, as well as the showers for use after swimming in the built-in heated cement pool. There were a couple of dorms, a chicken coop that had been converted into a boys' dorm and another small house where the staff lived.

I remember the drive up like it was yesterday. Along the way we spotted cattle, contained by a fence on the back roads. We stopped to look at them. They were curious creatures, and they came right up to the fence. I was thrilled at being able to pet a cow for the first time.

When we got to the camp, my father parked the car in a small circular area between the barn and the main house. "Eddie" (Mr. Madden) was sitting off to the side of this circle, on a lawn chair under a small tree between the house and the two dorms. Standing about 45 degrees over from him, almost right in front of the rec hall, was a kid, several years older than me. For the sake of conversation, let's call him Tom. Tom was the boy who would continue the tradition of me having a bully at camp. It seemed I was meant to have one no matter where I would go.

Madden Farm, or as it is known today, the Edward J. Madden Open Hearts Camp, was more akin to staying at your aunt and uncle's home than at a camp. We were allowed into the main house to eat, but access to the rest of the house was somewhat restricted. Overall, the farm felt more like a private home than it did a camp.

It didn't take very long at all for me to realize that *Yes, all the kids wore scars on their chests.* Most had a scar that either ran vertically or horizontally on their chests and some had scars that started on their chests but curved around onto their sides and ended up short of mid-back. I'd never seen that before. What I didn't see was anyone with *two* scars. I was the only one with that distinction. Finally, I'd found myself in a place where I did not have wear a tee shirt to go swimming.

Here was another first: As I hung around the other children I would hear them ask, "Where's Billy?" or "Where's Sally?" And then someone would answer, "Oh, they didn't make it, they died this winter," or other explanations of that order. We were, for the most part, all being stalked by death, and for us it was just another fact of life. It felt both bizarre and comforting at the same time that I was finally in a group where I wasn't the only one trying to elude death. That had been my unique "normal" for some years now, unique to me from every single person I knew in my life, and now my normal was, well, normal. In a strange way it took some of the pressure off, as if there was safety in numbers.

This was not a place where my strategy of cursing was going to work. This, as said before, was more like visiting a home rather than going to a sleep away camp. Mrs. Madden was a stickler for the social graces. We had to refer to them as *Mr.* and *Mrs.* and while at the dinner table, etiquette was to be observed. If one of us put our elbows on the table, Mrs. Madden would call out, "E-O-T!" which was shorthand for "Elbows off the table!" So, my cursing gambit certainly wouldn't fly here. Nor did I want it to, because in that setting even I thought it would have been just plain rude. After all, this was their home.

So, left without a tactic with which to defend myself, I fell victim to yet another camp bully. But at least it was never physical. "Tom" was the big man on campus; he was the most popular, the funniest, and this was his domain. If he didn't accept you, you weren't acceptable. But, unlike the other bullies, he didn't travel in a pack. In a sense, all the campers were in his pack, and once again I found myself to be one of the most unpopular kids. I say "one of" because there was another kid who was even more unpopular than me. Even *I* didn't like that kid. He was a smart-mouthed brat who went out of his way, it seemed, to *want* to make you dislike him. So, we did.

The Maddens were a wonderful older couple, most likely in their late sixties. I can still hear Mrs. Madden calling for her husband. "Eddieee," she would call out loudly whenever she needed him. "Eddieeeeeee!" They liked to interact with the children, but not too much. Mr. Madden had a habit that left what we called "minefields." He loved cigars. He had one in his mouth the very first time I saw him. But, being a heart patient, he wasn't allowed to smoke them. Instead he would keep the cigar in his mouth and, after a while, bite the saliva-soaked end off in his mouth, chew it for a short while and then spit it out onto the ground. Barefoot campers quickly learned to watch their steps anywhere Mr. Madden had been!

And then there were the paper fights. I think this was Mrs. Madden's idea, as I can't recall Mr. Madden playing in this game, but I could be wrong. For those fights, Mrs. Madden invited all the children into the house and all the rooms on the first floor, instead of just the kitchen and the dining area. We were, however, still forbidden to go upstairs. Each kid was given newspaper, which we rolled up into long hollow tubes, and we chased one another all over the house trying to hit each other, most often over the head! At one point, Mrs. Madden and I really got into it right at the foot of the staircase. *Whap! Whap! Whap!* We were really going at it; I still remember her great big smile and laughter as the two of use duked it out. We all had a ball. What generous people they were.

When Tom wasn't around, other kids would swim and play with me to an extent, but, as usual, I found myself alone most of the time. The camp was very unstructured, something I really liked, and there were very few group activities. I usually found myself down by the stream sitting on the bank below the little bridge that crossed it, fishing. Fishing was something I had become very good at since the camp where I had retaliated against the bully. At that camp with nothing more than a fish-hook and a few yards of line tied to a stick, I was able to out-fish every other boy at that camp in spite of their fancy rods and reels. So, it was that fishing again became my favorite pastime. The fishing wasn't all that good, but the stream was a wonderful place to explore. This was where I found my first crawfish and was able to watch insects that could walk on water.

There was no doubt things would have been different if "Tom" hadn't been there. His constant taunting made me a very unhappy camper.

36

At this juncture of my life, between the ages of nine to about twelve, my parents knew something empirically that I knew instinctively: Death—my death—was lurking just around the proverbial corner, hiding in the shadows and waiting for its chance to pounce and take my life. As my stay at Madden Farm had powerfully demonstrated, a lot of us survived our operations but didn't survive our childhoods. According to what the doctors told my parents, I was expected to be counted among those in that unfortunate group in the not-too-distant future. No one told me this then, but I knew it. *Knew it.* Years later, my mother told me that they had been told I wouldn't live past ten years. I was already several years past my expected expiration date and intended to continue that trend.

I was, of course, still bullying my heart, often every single day. But, as doctors and parents like to put it, I wasn't "thriving." I was still so thin I barely cast a shadow, and even if my arms and legs were strong for my size, my heart was still weak. But I kept at it. Whenever I felt that sensation in my chest that told me my heart wasn't feeling right, I would stop what I was doing and bully my heart. I was always either walking, swimming or riding my bike. Again, instinctively, I knew I had to do these things, and so I did them. Besides, I loved all those activities, and they all could be done alone.

On summer breaks from school, when not at camp, I'd leave my home in the morning and come back before suppertime. I'd spend the whole time exploring the plentiful woods that were part of my neighborhood. One summer I found a dense patch of growth within a short walking distance from my home. It was wild, but not exactly what you would call the woods. This lot was comprised of all sorts of dense brush, a lot of it with needle-sharp thorns, and, it seemed to me, to have a center, and by God, I was going to get in there. After a few days of trying to find a way in I finally did, and my efforts were richly rewarded. The brush finally opened into a large area, about a quarter of an acre or so. Inside I found a treasure trove of the biggest, sweetest blackberries you ever saw. Blackberries have always been my favorite berry and my explorations had led me to this patch with more berries than I could ever eat in the entire summer! It would be fair to say that on that first day in the blackberry patch, I almost ate myself sick. How wonderful a day that was!

Our street, a lane really, was being developed and the zoning required a minimum of two-acre lots. Ours was the fourth home on Orchard Lane. The lot next to us, three acres, was empty, one of my favorite playgrounds in its wild and undeveloped state with the lot next to it under construction.

I got the idea that other people might like blackberries as much as I did. I borrowed a plastic container from our kitchen, went to "my" patch, and filled the container to the brim, being very careful to fill it with beautiful, ripe berries. I then went to the construction site, let the workers try a few, and then sold them the rest for a dollar. Back then a dollar was actually worth something. An "endless" cup of coffee in a diner was five cents at that time. My allowance, which was earned by doing chores, was 25 cents. At the end of the day I would go back to the construction site, retrieve the container, wash it, and the next day repeat the process. It was this experience that taught me I didn't necessarily have to work for someone other than myself. My entrepreneurial fires had been ignited and have been burning brightly ever since.

But I discovered something even more important that summer.

On one particularly bright and beautiful late-summer morning I was sitting on my floor, Indian style, next to my bed under one of my windows. I had just finished a session of bullying my heart and happened to glance at my bare right foot. As I looked at it, a thought went through my mind and I, well, ran with it.

One day, I thought, *this foot is going to be dead – along with the rest of me.* I kept the focus on my foot. *It's going to be dead one day*, I kept thinking to myself over and over. The lesson that I would die, no matter how old I was or what condition my health was in, had been driven home with a sledgehammer that day when I was six and received Last Rites before my second operation. But this was different. *One day this foot will be DEAD.*

I kept repeating it over and over. *This foot will be dead. This foot is going to die. This foot will be dead.* Over and over and over. I thought, *well, when it's dead, there'll be a sock and shoe on it. It will be inside of a casket. It will be dark in there. The casket will be six feet under the ground.* Over and over. I wanted to feel the death. *What will it feel like?* Over and over, *this foot will be dead.* I wanted to *know.* Over and over and over again, trying to feel what death would feel like until finally, I went into a sort of trance where I felt nothing. Absolutely *nothing*. I was dead. Finally, I was satisfied because to my mind I now knew what death would feel like.

I called this technique "my dead foot," and practiced it about a quarter as much as I did bullying my heart. There was something that I knew, even at that age, that most people don't learn until their lives are mostly over. Not even my parents or my doctors knew it, I mean *knew* what I now knew. I *knew* I was going to die. *I KNEW IT!* Since the age of six I have known I would die, was convinced that one day my heart was going to attack and kill me, but now I didn't really care as much. I had faced death several times in my young life, had to fight it to stay alive, had to defend myself from it, go into mortal battle against it. But this was different. This time, I had called death out, told him I knew he was there, stared him square in the face, let him know he didn't frighten me. My dead foot had taught me that. I never felt so free, so in control, so powerful.

37

One of the kids from the Brookville school, let's call him Mark, came from a seriously wealthy family, and he was to become one of my nemesis in the seventh grade. It was late in the year, almost summer, and Mark and I had the same art class. One day the teacher decided we should have the class outdoors. The Locust Valley campus was large and beautiful, and the teacher had picked a treed area by a hill to conduct the class. For some reason, the teacher wasn't with us for the whole class and this was when Mark made his move. I don't remember the cause of this event, but I think Mark had taken something of mine and was taunting me to take it back. I gave chase and, of course, he could easily outrun me. So, there I was, in front of the entire class, running after Mark in a fruitless effort to catch him as he taunted and laughed to the great amusement of the entire seventh grade art class. God, how their collective laughter burned in my ears. What's worse was that at one point I lost my footing during the chase and rolled down the hill in front of the entire class, much to their great delight and Mark's triumphant laughter, which seemed to roar above the collective laughter of the class. It was absolutely humiliating.

A week or so later we were again in art class, and again I don't remember why, the teacher was gone. This was Mark's cue that it was safe to pick on me again. I was at my desk drawing with a pencil. Mark was standing behind me, taunting me to everyone's glee, and I started to smolder. The image of the incident on the hill was still fresh in my mind and the humiliation was still raw. My vision started to narrow into that black tunnel as it had once before, and that part of me once again just snapped. In one fluid move, I jumped up from my desk, pencil in hand, and spun on Mark. His hands came up, palms flat out in a gesture of "Hey, I was only kidding," and I took the pencil and stabbed him with it in the palm of his left hand. Dead center. I will never forget the look of shock on his face, the gasp that came from the entire class, and the surprise it was to me that I'd done such a thing.

Mark looked alternately at me and his hand in stunned disbelief. I looked at his hand with the same feeling. There was no one in that room more surprised than me. There wasn't any blood, there was no wound. I don't think it had even broken the skin, but it was the action I had taken that had him and everyone else stunned. The best way I can characterize his response would be, "What, you can't take a joke?" while I would say mine was, "This is only a joke to you."

He walked away from me in a room of stunned silence. I sat down and just stared at what I had been drawing, not really seeing it, not really seeing anything, still lost in the dark place I was just getting out of. Interestingly, he never told the teacher, I believe because he knew he deserved it. Fortunately, not long after the incident, the bell rang, and the class ended.

No one in that class ever said as much as a word to me again. It didn't matter. It was almost summer and a few weeks later I'd be returning to Madden Farm and Tom would take over where Mark had left off.

It never ended.

38

This was to be one of the most pivotal times of my young life, although I didn't know it yet. When this, my seventh-grade summer, was over, I was going to start in a new school, St. Dominic's High School in bucolic Oyster Bay. I was looking forward to it because I wouldn't know a single kid there. I knew it would be an opportunity for me to change and start with a clean slate. But I didn't have a strategy; didn't have a clue as how to do it. At least I would have a summer to work on it once I got past Madden Farm and Tom.

The first time my parents drove me up to Madden Farm, Tom was almost the first thing I saw. So, when we pulled up to the same little gravel circle, I scanned the area to see if maybe he'd be standing in that same spot again. But he wasn't.

I was resigned to the fact that that summer would be like the last. I'd have a small degree of acceptance when Tom wasn't around and none when he was. At those times, I'd just become Tom's personal toy. This would be a replay of last summer and the Brookville and Locust Valley schools, I figured. I'd be on my own and spend a lot of time by myself at the creek fishing. The rest I'd just have to endure.

As each of us swung our separate doors open, the Maddens came to greet us. My mother and father received a warm welcome from them, as did I. However, as the pleasantries continued, and the car was unloaded, I kept nervously scanning for Tom.

I don't remember who it was I asked or even if I'd asked, nor who had told me, or exactly when, but somewhere between ten minutes and an hour after arriving I was told that Tom had died.

Think of me what you will but my true, first reaction to the news was that my heart did a little jump of joy. That was it; that was my first reaction. A moment or two later it sunk in that I was joyful that he wouldn't be there, and that it was too bad it was because of his death rather than because of some other reason preventing him from attending camp that summer. That moment of joy cost me, as did the realization that my reaction was inappropriate. But part of me was glad that he had died. I admit it. Part of me was glad. I almost couldn't help it. Why not? I hated him. He'd done no actual physical harm to me, but he had caused me to live in fear instead of enjoying my vacation as the other campers had. I'd had nightmares because of and about him. He was the reason I dreaded going back to camp. At home, I lay awake at nights in fear of what camp was going to be like that summer because of him. He continued the long string of medical procedures and bullies that had me in a constant state of shame and without a drop of self-worth. He thought it was fun to humiliate people in front of others. He, like all the rest, thought it was just fine to make himself big by making someone else small, someone who had never done anything wrong to him, ever. He made my life hell, and yet, somehow, while he was doing that he was the favorite of everyone, including the counselors and the Maddens. I never understood that. It's never made sense to me how it was that the cruel boys, the bullies, the worthless cowards, were always everyone's favorite. It wasn't until very recently that I've finally come to terms with my conflicted feelings about Tom's death and my reactions to it. It had haunted me for a long time. But the bottom line was that his death and that summer at Madden Farm gave me the opportunity to re-invent myself, to leave the old Steven behind, the Steven who has a heart problem and was unpopular and the target of bullies. The Steven whose shame and worthlessness I dragged around and could be seen by everyone. The Steven who was responsible for all the negative things and dynamics in my family. The Steven who was at fault for all of it. This was my chance and I was going to take it. I'm quite certain it wouldn't have happened if Tom hadn't died. And that's the God's honest truth.

39

I quickly realized I now had two opportunities in front of me, and in a way, each depended on the other. I already knew I had the opportunity of a re-start with the advent of entering a completely new school in September. But I had thought I'd have to endure camp and Tom first, and then try to think up a new strategy after camp before starting at the new school. Things seemed to have shifted in my favor. I had a chance to both enjoy that session at Madden Farm and do a dry-run of the new me at the same time.

I thought about who I was at the time, and more importantly, how I was perceived by others. Who was I? I was this person who deeply believed—and to a large extent still do as of this writing—that everything negative in my life was my fault and, worse, that all those things happened to me *because I deserved it.* That's why I was always bullied; all you had to do was look at me and know I deserved it. All you had to do was *look* at me and know I wasn't any good. "I'm no good and I deserve it" were the two key themes of my life. Okay, that was who I was.

How was I perceived? I was the skinny, sick and weak kid. I almost never said anything, my eyes and head were always down, and, as a friend once told me, I looked as if there were rain clouds above my head all the time. Bad luck was my shadow. I always kept my eyes focused a few inches in front of my feet and I never looked anyone in the eye. I was afraid that if I looked someone in the eye, in that moment they'd know how worthless I was, how I was no good, how I deserved to have bad things happen to me.

This is a good place to point something out. I almost never spoke in school, or at a hospital, but at home I was a regular chatterbox. I drove my parents nuts with my barrages of constant questions and tendency to rattle on. And while it is true that I never cried a single tear in the hospital or at home for my heart troubles or the incredible pain I'd gone through, at home I cried about everything else. It took me years to figure out that while I was *dissociating* by hiding in my cave or riding my seagull, the pain that I thought I didn't feel, the fear, the *terror* that I experienced but never acknowledged, had to go somewhere. So, while I was busy being a good boy who could watch other children be taken to their deaths, I waited for them to come for me next. And while I endured genuine agony multiple times and yet never reacted to it, all of that emotional and physical pain was going somewhere, and that *somewhere* had to vent. My talking and crying became that vent. It took me most of my life before I figured this out, but what surprised me once I did was that my parents never figured it out either. I think they were so busy pretending I was normal that it never came into view for them.

The upshot of all this venting behavior was that I created more resentment in my siblings and father as my mother became more and more protective of me, which was the exact opposite of what I wanted. I was just a terrified and hurting little boy and no one ever figured it out.

Sure, my brothers picked on me, but I was their little brother, and I assume some of that was natural. But there was also resentment, which meant I had no safe place. At school it was bullies, and when I came home, I'd often got more of the same, although usually not to the same degree. So, it was either making models, sitting under my dad's piano, or in the refuge of my mother where I could feel things were safe. Or as safe as they could feel for me.

Or I could play with my sister, Neiani, which we did a lot. We made up games that included my car models and make-believe families whose roles we would play, and we'd sit on the floor of my room playing for hours. The bottom line when it came to my brothers and sister was, adopted or not, they were my brothers and sister and I always loved them as such. Deeply. As far as I was concerned, then and now, they were and are, blood. I have many wonderful memories with them and I hold those memories dearly.

So, after I'd taken this inventory of my life, I had to decide who I was going to be.

The answer came to me quickly. After some thought I determined all I had to do was turn everything 180 degrees around. I was extremely shy, so now I'd be the opposite. I would become the extrovert. I never spoke outside of the home; well, those days were over. I knew I could make people laugh, so I'd become the comedian. I'd do my best to keep my head up and look others in the eyes, but I didn't master that one until I was in my thirties. But I did a better job of it. I was always sad, but now I was going to always be happy, even if it was a front and I was still sad and insecure inside. I would no longer look beaten down. I would look as if life was okay with me and that I was okay with it.

I also looked at what little had worked in my life before. I'd beaten-up a bully at Camp Molloy. I kept bullies away with cursing at Boy Scout camp, and the fact that I still had serious heart troubles hadn't kept me from winning that canoe race. *really*, I thought to myself, *I was stronger than I thought, including the fact that I was still alive in spite of the fact that I was passed my "due date."* That made me realize I had strength enough to do this. I found those thoughts to be bracing.

No one realized more than myself that this would be an act, a costume of my own imagination that I would cloak myself with, but, *damn it*, it was this or the life I'd been living. Believe me, I was done with that. And no matter how difficult it was going to be, no matter how hard it would be for me to be the extrovert in the group, the one who cracked the jokes, the one who wouldn't hesitate to introduce himself to one person or a group, *I was going to do this*.

And, so I did.

40

There was no transition, no gingerly dipping a toe in the water or holding a wet finger to the social winds. I simply jumped in with both feet. I was once told that the word *decide* meant "to cut off from everything else," so once the decision was made on who the new me was going to be, my outward personality changed at the speed of a finger snap. This didn't surprise me because I knew it was the only way that this could work; all or nothing. Well, I'd already had a lifetime of nothing, leaving me with the only choice that I had had to go for it all. It simply made sense. I knew I'd make mistakes along the way, but when I did I would determine what they were and adjust accordingly. So, I held my nose, closed my eyes, and jumped into what were for me strange and unchartered waters, and as I did I cut everything else off and left it on the shore behind me.

Earlier that year I had started to study the electric guitar. I brought my metal-flake red guitar with me to camp. I wasn't very good at it; in truth, I was terrible. I had just started lessons but bringing the guitar with me that summer had been a good idea. Apparently, it increased my "cool factor" just by having it there, and since I didn't have an amplifier with me the fact that I could barely play went just about un-noticed. But it helped because some of the kids told other kids that I had it, and, thank God, that apparently was enough.

I was a pretty quick thinker, as well as being extremely observant, and that helped me in becoming the camp comedian. I discovered that I very much enjoyed making others laugh and not just because it bolstered my popularity, which was rising exponentially. It made me feel good to make others feel good. I downright enjoyed it.

Well, my plan was a success, at least outwardly. I make that distinction because every time I did or said something, I was in an internal near-panic that it would be wrong, in panic that whomever it was I was dealing with would discover I was "no good inside" and now, worse, a fraud to boot. I came off as confident. It's like sincerity; it's easy once you know how to fake it, as the old joke goes. But confident was the very last thing I was. I turned all my turmoil entirely inward, and even more than before, I was always afraid, always dreading the inevitable next thing that would hit me with my heart or, and I think I feared this more, the discovery that I was a fraud. I didn't get any kind of a handle on that until just a few years ago.

Nevertheless, I was popular for the first time in my life—with both the boys *and* the girls—and that was all I cared about. Mrs. Madden, however, did not like the new me. I'd become a little too wild for her taste and, like I said, I jumped into this new character headlong. I was just taking wild guesses at what my behavior should be, the fact it rubbed her the wrong way was just going to have to be ignored. There was no going back. If Mrs. Madden didn't like it, her approval was going to have to be a casualty in my new battle. I didn't like it, but I was in the place that I couldn't, or more accurately, didn't know how to rectify it without destroying what was working well for me. That genuinely upset me and her looks of disapproval cut me deeply, hurt the me that was still there hidden under my new cloak, made me even more insecure. But for the first time in my life I was making friends, having fun, and most importantly, being allowed to be part of a group, even, to my great surprise, to be one of the leaders. So, I kept my head down and continued on into the unknown fray.

One of the kids I made friends with was named Justo Martinez, a Hispanic boy from Brooklyn. We remained friends for years and then, sadly, lost touch. I've been trying to find him for a long, long time, but to no avail. I remade contact with another of my friends from the farm a couple of years ago, and she thinks he might not be with us anymore. I hope she's wrong. I used his real name in the hopes that this will help us to re-connect somehow. Justo, I think of you often.

My experiment had been a great success; my trial run for who I should be when I got to St. Dominic's was complete. There were holes in my new persona. I'd have to be on the watch for them and plug them when I could, but for the first time in my life I was looking forward to going to school.

41

For the rest of that summer I no longer felt as if I had to hide as much as I used to. The move to Brookville and the class-consciousness of the kids there had made me even more ostracized than I'd been in Malverne. At the same time, it gave me much larger areas to explore. There were fields, woods and the occasional new house going up in the area for me to investigate. Sometimes, though, I didn't want to explore. I just wanted to be alone and quiet. Before that second summer I had two favorite hiding spots, both of which were on our three-acre property. Going from the front to the back, our parcel started with a large lawn, (about half an acre) the house, my father's attached studio, the pool and cabanas, a lightly wooded area, and thick trees and brush for maybe the last quarter acre. Next to us was an empty lot that would be developed, but it added three acres of wild fields.

My parents were still worried about my past "due date," but I was full of energy. I think both them and I thought my frequent excursions from the house were healthy for me. I had put the physical problems I suffered in the back of my mind as best I could, which wasn't easy with the hot pink scars I'd been branded with. But I did my best and discovered hiding did a couple of things for me. First, it would quiet my mind. Second, if I was hiding, the fact that I was alone was okay. And third, I liked having places no one else knew about, secret places that were mine, although I ended up showing both of them to Neiani. I just never told her I hid in them. I shared them with her so we could play. She didn't know I went to them by myself as often as I did.

The first hiding place was in plain sight: a large, gorgeous maple tree that stood off a back corner of our house, between the house, the pool and the patio. It had a low enough branch for me to mount and then a series of branches that might as well have been a ladder.

About mid-point in this tree formed a crotch, with two strong branches going out from the bottom and the trunk splitting in two and traveling upward from there. The first time I found that spot it felt like it had been created just for me. I could put my feet on the two branches, lean back against the divided trunk, and, I swear, it felt as if the tree were hugging me. It fit my butt and back perfectly, so much so that I napped there–about 15 feet above the ground. On more than one occasion I'd have gone into my tree and then Mom and Dad would go to sit on the patio to enjoy afternoon coffee. Even if they were speaking in low voices, I could hear them most of the time. I used to delight when one or the other of them would ask, "Where's Steven?"

"*I'm right here!*" I'd say to myself.

The other hiding place was at the back of the property. We were bordered by Orchard Lane in the front and Northern Boulevard (Rt. 25A) in the back, a moderately busy four-lane without streetlights or sidewalks. One day, while digging around back there looking for who knows what, I found a drainage pipe that ran under Northern Boulevard to the property across the street. I was just small enough to fit without a problem. Today that would not be the case! That was something else I liked about it: not too many could follow me in there. So, after getting in the pipe far enough to get a good look for raccoons or debris, of which there was none of either, I made the underground journey to the other side of Northern Boulevard.

The other side was a gentleman's farm, lush grass and trees and a BULL! With HORNS! I don't think he liked me, because he charged at me. I dove for the pipe, got back in time and belly-crawled back to our side. Man, I thought that was a hoot! A real adventure.

This became my other nap place, but more usually just a place I liked to visit and relax in. I liked going there for several reasons. First, no one knew about it but me for a long time, until I told Neiani about it. Second, *I was under a road!* I would try to position myself so I'd be under a lane, not the center where no cars were. I'd lay there, two or three feet below the pavement, wondering what kinds of cars and trucks were passing directly over me, amazed at how I didn't feel or hear them as they did. And, just as it was when sleeping in my tree, there was some-thing exciting about it, a whiff of danger, if you will. But this time the danger was under my control, and I think, in a small way, it was *me* challenging death. This was only the beginning of that kind of behavior.

I'd also wonder, *what would happen to me if I died in here?* They'd never find me. It'd be years later, I'd think, when my bones were found accidentally and the mystery of, "Whatever happened to that little heart kid?" would be solved. I couldn't tell you exactly why, but that thought always gave me a thrill and made me smile. Again, I think that's because death would've been under my terms.

I loved those two spots, but after that second summer at Madden Farm, while I would still occasionally climb that maple just for the fun of it, I never felt the need to hide in either the tree or the under highway again.

42

Everything about St. Dominic's was a different experience from any other school I'd ever attended. First, and foremost, it was a Catholic school and the majority of my teachers would be nuns. Second, I had to wear the school uniform to class: dress pants, a white shirt and a school tie. The girls had to wear white blouses and a school skirt of a certain length—and no shorter!

There were about 40 children in my eighth-grade class, and believe me, that many students were not a problem. Maybe that was because there was discipline in those days. I had a friend I'll speak about in a moment whose entire pre-college education took place at St Dom's. I only had two years and one day there, all the rest of my schooling was public. There is no doubt about which of us received the superior education.

On my first day, I slipped a note to a boy a couple desks to the left and in front of me. The note read, DO YOU WANT TO BE IN MY BAND? Joe and I are still friends today. I'd already made my first inroad and all it took was for me to screw up all the courage I could muster to write and pass that note.

Earlier that summer or the one before, I can't remember which, my oldest brother, Peter, came home on leave from the Air Force. While in the Air Force, he'd taken up karate. One afternoon he showed me how to defend myself from a dog attack, which, fortuitously, came in handy when, as it happened, I was attacked by a large Standard Poodle that weighed about three-quarters of what I did at the time.

I'd had dogs all my life since the day I was born. At that time, we had three: a large, 100- pound German Shepherd named Pepper, a 50-pound mutt named Ginger, and my mother's Chihuahua, Chico. Point being, I knew when a dog was running over to play or was in an attack mode. That dog was attacking. There was no doubt. As the dog came charging at me, I heard Peter's instructions in my head clearly: *Don't run, it turns you into prey. Face the dog head on, stand your ground and lift your arm so as to cross your face, about a foot forward of your chin. This is what the dog will jump for, as it is the closest target you offer, and they like to go for the throat in the first place. When the dog leaps for your arm, before his mouth can get to your arm, bring your knee up as quickly and strongly as you can, kicking it in the chest and knocking the wind out of him. Then get away.*

I followed these instructions to the letter and left a dog almost as big as me on the side of the road where he had jumped for me, completely knocked out of breath but basically unhurt. I only mention this because some other things Peter taught me would come in just as handily the next time a dog, this time much bigger than me, jumped me inside St. Dominic's itself.

I spent the eighth and ninth grades and one day of tenth at St. Dominic's. My friendship with Joe brought me into his already established circle of friends and eighth grade was the first time I had a "normal" experience in a school.

In the beginning of ninth grade, the new school year was maybe a week old when I had attracted the attention of this kid who was to be my next and last bully. Of course, he was much bigger than me. Our class had gone to the school basement where the cafeteria was to have lunch. We were gathered near the stairwell waiting for the place to open when new-kid came up to me and, with what started as taunts, quickly became challenging shoves. You know, the kind that mean, "So, what are you gonna do about it?" Of course, most of the class was watching. I knew that this had become the make-or-break moment, not just for this school, but for the rest of my life. This was my first serious challenge for the new me and I had to answer it. Almost instantly, I knew just what I was going to do about it. But instead of my reaction coming from an almost uncontrollable dark rage, this time it came from a cool, calculated summation of the situation based on what I'd learned from dealing with bullies in the past and my recent lessons from Peter.

His back was to the wall about four feet behind him. He shoved me again, which was exactly what I needed, because that gave me the room to mount my defense. As I did in Camp Molloy, I put my head down and charged. Shocked surprise registered on his face. I don't think it ever entered his mind that someone half his size would defend themselves against him. I bet it never happened before. Well, things change, don't they?

My shoulder rammed into him and I drove him back, hard, into the cinder block wall behind him. When his back hit the wall, his head followed with what was a stunning blow. That was my part; now came Peter's. As soon as his head hit the wall, my knee came up with everything I had. You can guess where I was aiming for, and, fortunately, my aim was perfect.

This caused him to bend at the waist, mouth wide open from the blooming pain being transmitted from his loins, hands cupping his legacy makers. I knitted my two hands together into a tight ball and brought them up from underneath in a reverse hammer blow. I connected with his open jaw, snapping his mouth shut with an audible sound of his teeth cracking together, his head now having been snapped up from the result of the hit, and with what was the combination of a moan and a sigh, he slid down along the wall until his butt hit the floor and his legs splayed forward; he just sat, groaning and half out of it. There was no doubt about it, he was in a dazed state. The circle of kids who witnessed this were slack-jawed, and sticking to my new persona, Joe, another friend, and I walked away as if nothing big had happened.

But something big did happen. No one at that school ever thought I was fodder for a bully again. Not only that, no one ever tried to bully me again, *ever*. I think the thing that attracted bullies to me was destroyed that day, and for the rest of my life I haven't had to absorb or defend myself from a bully since.

To this day, I'm not exactly sure how that worked because I was a terrified little kid under that cloak, but it did. And that was all that mattered, the new-me strategy was working perfectly.

43

I was making friends, hung out with groups of boys, and had the best summer of my life in eighth grade, and there was no summer camp that year or any year after, for that matter. Ninth grade was similar but, unbeknownst to me, I was also gliding downhill to my next medical emergency.

At this juncture in the story, it's important that I point something out. I have all the medical records, and more, for the two months I'd spent in St. Francis Hospital. They total somewhere around 50 pages. Yes, that's correct, around 50 pages. My current hospital records are in four-inch binders, at least three of them that I've seen, but it could be even more than that. I don't know. But I do know that when I had my first two operations, the government wasn't involved in medicine *at all*. We used to have a family doctor who made house calls, who would base his billing on a patient's ability to pay. Those who could afford it would be billed more and poorer patients less, if at all. That's the way it was back then, everything was between the patient and the doctor.

I remember him lamenting to my mother that he could no longer do that type of billing because Medicare or Medicaid made that illegal. *He could go to jail if he billed a poorer person at a lower rate!* I also heard him say he didn't know how much longer he would be able to make house calls. Not long after that he didn't come to our house anymore. Now, I don't know the exact reason for that, but I do know he was forced, let me say that again, *forced*, to change the way he practiced medicine. I must have been ten or eleven when this happened, but even then I didn't understand how the government could do that. That seemed to be no different than the way bullies had treated me. It made me wonder how the government had become a bully, too.

More important to this story is the part about the records. From here in, I'm working off my memory and the accounts of others. I apologize if I get some small detail wrong here or there. But I can promise you whatever I write from this point on, as well as what has already been written, I believe to be factually true. At least, factually true to me. I'm telling you exactly how I remember it, and I won't say anything for portions that I can't recall. Although, to tell you the truth, I can't imagine what that might be. So, for the eighth and ninth grade I'm a pretty happy child—kind of.

My parents' marriage had been dissolving for more than a decade and by now all the ties that once bound them had melted into an ugly, slobbering monster that stained the entire household with its bitter residue. Peter had already left for good when he joined the Air Force. Later, Michael will have gotten himself declared an emancipated minor. At the beginning of this dissolution, Michael was attending La Salle Military Academy, a private school. After that, he'd be off to college (Rutgers in New Jersey). Neiani and I were left home with my mother and my father's occasional visits. He hadn't left the home yet, but he never seemed to be there, either. I also remember occasions where Neiani and I were pressed to a wall listening, while my parents fought in another room. It was horrible. I recall how shaken it made us to hear those fights.

I vividly remember one fight where my father wanted to pull Michael from La Salle. My father had made some serious investment mistakes, and everything was gone. We weren't out of the house yet, but that was gone, too.

This fight was as bad as any of them ever were with my mother screaming at my father so loudly, so defiantly, that Michael should stay at La Salle. (He did, and it helped him to launch a successful career.) What I always liked about this was that she fought as hard for him as she ever did for me. It somehow made me feel a little less guilty.

The divorce finally came during my ninth-grade summer, ironically on the twenty-third anniversary of their marriage. How's that for irony? Neiani had decided to move in with my father and I stayed with Mom. We rattled around in that huge house set on three acres with a 52- foot-long pool and two out-buildings for several months. All maintenance fell to me, and I was overwhelmed by it. Soon, the grounds and pool fell into disarray. Then the strangers came, people who wanted to see if that was the house for them. They looked in my room and my closet, as well as the rest of the house, and every time people came to look I felt that my world was being invaded and falling apart more and more; nowhere to feel safe. A re-occurring theme in my life.

The house was sold, there was almost no equity left, and we moved to Port Washington on Long Island's North Shore with no money. Mom and I were dead broke. While still in Brookville, my mother was forced to go back to working as a nurse, but it wasn't enough. Really, we were broke, and my father started playing games with alimony (beginning with not paying it) and illegally saddling my mother with a huge part of his debt. I was in court watching when the judge asked my mother if she wanted to prosecute my father for perjury. The judge wanted to throw my father in jail then and there. Without putting too fine a point on it, the judge was outraged. Absolutely outraged. My mother declined, but our situation didn't improve.

Here's an example of how things were before we went to court. We were set to move to Port Washington in October. I was going to continue school at St. Dominic's until then. On the first day of school, grades nine to twelve were assembled in the auditorium, which was also the basketball court when configured as such for orientation. Just before orientation was completed, my name was called out in front of the entire high school. Joe and I were sitting next to each other, as always. I got up, made my way down the bleachers to the nun who was waiting for me. I was escorted to the principal's office where I was informed my tuition hadn't been paid and I had to go home.

You can imagine my mother's reaction to this. She was under the impression that my father had paid it. He refused to pay the tuition, and the school refused to let me stay for the six or seven weeks until we moved. No matter how many phone calls my mother made or how much she pleaded, St. Dom's wouldn't relent. I had to be re-enrolled in Locust Valley High School once again. Locust Valley was where I defended myself in art class. As you would expect, this was far from an ideal situation for me on several different levels.

So, I was forced to leave the first school where I had friends and wasn't bullied and compelled to go back to the one that was the exact opposite. Luckily, that encounter with the bully in St. Dominick's really had changed me. Maybe some remembered the incident in art class, but whatever the reason, I was mostly left alone and found a small group I could hang with while my real friends were in a different school.

Finally, moving day arrived. Mom and I left a house that I loved to move into a home that could literally, and I mean literally, fit into the basement of the Brookville house with room to spare. Six days later, Pepper, our beautiful six-year-old German Shepherd, died suddenly in my arms in my new bedroom. A few days later, in middle October, I started the tenth grade at Paul D. Schreiber High School in Port Washington.

As I referenced earlier, while all this was going on something else started to happen. Towards the end of the ninth grade, I could detect a change in my heart. I can't quite remember how it first showed up, but I could feel it. By March of the tenth grade the situation had progressed into a life-threatening problem. It really did look like the doctor's prediction that I wouldn't make it out of my teens just might come true. Time to do battle. Again.

44

Socially, I did well at Schreiber. I made a lot of friends. Especially with a boy named David. I also came into my own with the fairer sex and dated and had a lot of friends who were girls.

But the heart.

I had this sense that I had to cram as much as I could into whatever time there was. Someone who was older had told me to enjoy my youth because it would be over in a blink. I took him at his word and tried to have as much fun as I could. I guess underneath it all one could say I was afraid for my life, and I guess that's true to a certain extent. But that's not the way I thought of things; not the way I operated. I just had this unshakeable belief that nothing was wrong with me—even when there was. This was just my "normal." As I did when I received Last Rites, there was a part of me that wouldn't allow the thinnest crack to appear in that foundation of belief that I believed then, as I do now, is what kept me alive.

So, I started with a new cardiologist, a young guy who was

probably twice my 16 years. We clicked immediately, and he quickly understood where I was coming from, what I'd already been through. He always spoke directly and honestly with me; nothing was ever sugarcoated. He had gathered correctly that was the way I needed to be dealt with, that that was the way I defended myself from my physical problems. Besides, by that time my mother was his office nurse and he also gathered, correctly, she'd tell me anyway.

We're middle tenth grade here. The news the doctor had for me was not good and even kind of bizarre to boot.

My resting heart rate was an astonishing 172. You read that correctly: 172.

Once, when he had me exercise strenuously, it brought my rate up to 178. After several other tests, he'd figured it all out. He sat me down in the exam room and gave me the news. I had maybe a year to live before my heart tore itself apart. It wasn't beating as much as it was fluttering. He wasn't sure if that was some kind of disease process or, more than likely, the heart rate center of my heart—a little node we all have—had been damaged during the second operation when I was six. This is the part of the heart that connects to the brain. It's how your heart knows that a bear is chasing you and that it had better speed up *now*. He thought that would be the most likely culprit. At some point in the future I would have to go to the hospital so we could find out exactly what was wrong. But we were going to wait a little bit. I think he thought it might resolve itself on its own, but that is a pure guess on my part.

That night, my mother and I had a short but serious conversation on what I had been told. She confirmed it all, and as it was the way we handled those things, we pretended nothing had happened. We never spoke about it again for almost a year.

A year. A year to live. But, like I said, somewhere deep inside me wouldn't believe it. *I* absolutely wouldn't allow myself to believe it.

What was I supposed to do with that information? I don't know if my father was told, but I know my siblings weren't. My mother and I had decided to keep that one to ourselves. And I decided to keep it from my friends as well. We both agreed that would be the best course of action in the situation.

The last thing I wanted was to tell Joe, David or anyone else for that matter that I might only have a year or so. The thing I feared the most, the thing I most didn't want to see, was the look in their eyes, that flash of pity when they might on occasion think I could be dead soon. I don't think I could've taken it. I also didn't want to have to talk about it. All of that: the looks, the talking, would only make me weaker. And I didn't need *that*. What I needed was fun and distraction.

There were three distinct groups in my high school: the jocks, the hippies and the gear heads, also known as greasers. Among the friends I made, a bunch of them were gear heads. I was the only long-hair in the group. But our love of cars, muscle cars in particular, was enough of an equalizer. This was the muscle car era. I'd go riding with them every Friday night and sometimes Saturday nights looking for a street race. During the summer, it was most nights. We always found at least one a night. Man, I have never tired of acceleration. I love it. I love it just as much now—brutal, throw-you-into-your-seatback and pin-you-there acceleration. I was always a car guy, and even if I was still too young to drive, those cars just sealed the deal for me. A few of those cars were monsters; unbelievably powerful, hopped-up monsters. My friend Les' car was never beat that I know of. And those guys were good, loyal friends, too.

There was a small cottage colony in Port Washington at the time called, well, The Colony. These were summer cottages built into a steep hill overlooking Roslyn Harbor and Bar Beach. When we were done racing and cruising, this is where we'd go. With a couple of six-packs in hand, we'd walk to the beach, sometimes build a fire, shoot the bull, talk about cars and girls and have a couple of beers. They didn't seem to mind that I didn't particularly like beer and almost always didn't have any. If I did, I'd usually make one can of beer last all night.

I liked going there because a resident of The Colony named Harriet was also on the beach on those nights. Harriet and I developed a deep friendship. We felt like we'd always known each other. Old souls, or something like that. We're still friends, phone friends now, even though we haven't seen each other since we were 16.

One night, one of the last times I saw her, Harriet wanted to read my palm. I'd seen her do it with others and she sure did seem to have some type of gift. She took my hand, the one and only time we'd ever touched, and started to read. When she got to my lifeline she looked confused and said I had the most inter-rupted lifeline she had ever seen. Then suddenly, with a quick catch of her breath, she said I was in immediate danger and that I could die well within the year. She didn't say I *would* but there was a good chance I *could*. She looked at me with an expression that fluctuated between total shock and sadness.

I had told no one. *No one!* I tried to act as nonchalant as possible, tried to brush it off. But she wasn't buying it. Her expression didn't change, and I knew that she knew. She knew I knew she knew, too, and that added up to an absolute *she knows*. Still, I pretended, but nothing during that year, nothing I'd been told about my heart, roiled me the way that moment had.

I didn't allow it to last for long. I had to get back to my belief system, but the bottom line was I had been shaken. Thoroughly shaken.

45

Summer ended, and I started the eleventh grade. Time was coming, and fairly soon, that I'd have to go to the hospital, but I wasn't thinking about it almost at all. In reality, not at all. I didn't keep it in my head; I just had no room in my life for thoughts of death.

My mother and I had a deep understanding of each other. In spite of all of our fights, of which there were many, we both knew at the most elemental level that we had each other's backs. My grades were good, but girls and friends were much more important to me at that point, and Mom "got it." There was that "condition" we wouldn't talk about, and we both knew school wasn't the end-all to us that it might be to others who had less pressing issues to deal with. She just got it. I'd stopped taking the bus to school almost as soon as I'd started at Schreiber, hitch-hiking my way to and from there instead. I was pretty much on my own schedule. I started to cut classes or school altogether while maintaining good grades, always having to ask for a note so I wouldn't get in trouble. So, Mom and I made a deal: As long as my grades continued to be good, I could write my own notes for being late or missing school the previous day. My forgery of my mother's signature was *excellent*. So, that's what I did.

Well, as luck would have it, one day I was caught writing an excuse note for my absence of the previous day by my homeroom teacher. I was leaning against a locker in the hall writing the note when she caught me. She was triumphant and had a satisfied sneer as she told me to stay where I was. She walked across the hall to call a school disciplinarian from the classroom phone. I could only imagine his glee on hearing my current situation: *Caught red handed! Got you! Finally!* I was sure I had just made his day. I could feel his delight coming though the phone line from across the hall. I was told to report to his office post-haste.

Let's just say that that man and I had a history. In the tenth grade I had been dating a girl whose parents didn't like me one bit. Part of it was because I was Italian, part because my mother was divorced, and part because my hair was a little long, about the same length the Beatles wore when they first came here. They were old-fashioned, all capital letters WASPS. The combination made me radioactive to them. They had called on this man to help me see the error of my ways for dating their daughter. One day while standing on the front steps of the school he had threatened me as to what would happen if I continued to date her. It didn't work, of course, and because of that the guy still had it in for me. My mother hadn't forgotten that episode, which she considered an abuse of power when he stuck his nose into what was personal, not school, business. It really steamed her.

I sat calmly in his office, longish hair and all, while he licked his chops. He asked me if I had an explanation. I calmly told him, why yes, I did: My mother had written the note. I'd finished the note, signature and all, while leaning against another locker, on my way down to his office.

"What? You were caught red handed writing the note! Mrs. Busybody saw you writing it!"

"No, my mother wrote the note."

"*Really?*"

"Really."

"So why don't we call her and find out?"

"She's not home, she's at work."

"You wouldn't happen to know the number, would you?"

"Why, *sure.*"

I gave it to him. I don't think I ever saw anyone dial a phone with as much determination.

"Hello, Mrs. Taibbi, this is Mr. Drunk with Power at Schreiber. I have your son here and he was caught writing an excuse note...."

You have to love my mother. She was often surprisingly cool. She cut him off, told him she had written the note and that if he wouldn't mind (and as snippily as she could) asked for him to please not call her at work for unimportant matters. Then she hung up. The look on his face—I wish I could describe it, but he was totally deflated and dumbfounded, to say the least. I stood up, took the note so I could give it back to Mrs. Busybody, asked if there was anything else, and walked out. Back in homeroom, I handed the note back to a flabbergasted Mrs. Busybody. Priceless.

Of course, both my mother and I were thrilled we'd knocked the snot out of that self-important little man, but really something bigger had taken place. It was our un-acknowledged acknowledgement that our lives were different, and only we knew what made that difference. It was both of us telling me: Have fun and go live.

I didn't waste any of it.

46

L ate April came as did the time I had to go to the hospital; this time Long Island Jewish Hospital, in Great Neck. None of my friends, including my best friends Joe, David and Concetta, aka Chet, or Bean, as I called her, knew anything more than that I was going in for a standard test. I was able to pass this fiction off to one and all.

I was sixteen, a week or so from seventeen. I was going to LIJ to get a catheterization to see if they could determine what was wrong, but unlike when I was five and six, there would be no incision in the groin, no four-inch scars in the area of my all-time favorite muscle. Medicine had advanced a great deal since then. Instead, they would use a device to puncture their way into my artery, and thread a tube through the collar that made the puncture.

Now, compared to today, the size of the tubing to be used was the size of a garden hose, and the copper-colored collar looked huge to me. Let me describe it to you. It was basically a metal tube several inches long, under a quarter of an inch in diameter, with a circular flange that grew out of the upper third of the tubing with an edge, or lip, around that. That was it. They also had to make an incision in the crook of my right elbow, of about an inch and a half, and that was its own trip.

You have to be awake during a cardiac catheterization because they ask you to hold your breath at certain times. They do give you a mild sedative, mostly to calm you, but certainly not enough to put you to sleep. For the incision in my arm, I was given a local. It's always been funny to me that a local anesthetic injection should hurt. Just one of those ironies. I've been given the local, and the doctor doing this part of the procedure has to give me more because the incision he is creating is hurting me, although it's not supposed to by that point. That's when I heard the doctor say what every comedian says you don't want to hear your doctor say: "Uh oh." *Uh oh?* The unusual architecture of my venous system is part of my original birth defects. I've been told I have "friable" veins. In any case, in this situation, it meant that my vein was deeper than the average person's. That meant a local couldn't reach to the depth needed. Did I think I could hang on while he continued to cut? Well, sure. Why not? *What am I supposed to say? No?* They'd continue anyway.

You know, many times in my life I've been told that I'm brave. Brave? Can we talk about brave here, because that situation couched the subject perfectly? What else are you going to do? They strap you to a table. You've surrendered all of your will, your power, your *dignity and your life,* to strangers wearing gowns and masks who you've never met. You will never even know what they look like. Brave? Again, *what else are you going to do*—flail and scream? Makes no sense. You just do what you have to do if you want to stay alive. So, I clenched my teeth while he did what he had to do. I guess, in the end, that's what both of us did.

With that part of the procedure finished, it was time for the actual catheterization.

I can't express how sinister this simple device looked. Then the doctor—not my doctor, he wasn't there, but the cath doc, asked if I was ready. Yes. And this I will never, ever forget. The doctor, with the device in the middle of balled fists, places the cath over the spot on my groin he wanted, and then, while not moving the device from its placement, either jumped up a couple of inches or just raised himself on his toe tips and drove that tube in with a great deal of force. *Oh, MOTHER OF HOLYCRAP, DID THAT HURT!* For weeks after I had nightmares about that moment. I would involuntarily have flashbacks during the day as well. After a while, the flashbacks and the nightmares receded, but that moment is laser-burned into my memory, and whenever I give it thought, such as now, I can see the whole scene as if it just happened ten seconds ago.

The cath confirmed there was no disease process or other physical anomaly causing the problem, which left the theory of the damaged heart rate center. They did what was, I believe, the only thing left to do in the medical arsenal of the times. They were going to do a cardio version or *cardio vert*, as it's more popularly known, on me. That's fancy doctor talk for *electrocution*. No kidding. The doctor explained what was going to happen and what they *hoped* would happen, along with what they hoped *wouldn't* happen. I was to make an informed decision, but to be truthful because I was a minor my decision may not have counted at all. But I'm grateful I was made a part of the process. Really, that's always better, at least for me. The doctor explained they were going to knock me out, now required because a local wouldn't be enough, put a metal plate on my back, and another on my chest. Then they would zap me with the purpose of stopping my heart. No, that irony did not escape me. Then they would wait a little bit, but not so long as to cause brain damage—although my wife swears they *did* wait too long —and then zap me again, this time to restart the heart. The thinking was this would give the heart and brain a chance to re-connect and thus restore regulation of the heart.

On the downside was the possibility of brain damage and the off, you know, slight, teeny-tiny, highly improbable chance the heart wouldn't restart.

Oh, yeah, okay. Sure, let's do it.

As you have figured out by now, the heart did restart, and the heart-brain connection was restored. I came out of my induced sleep looking straight at a heart monitor. The heart rate was in the low 80's. I couldn't have been happier. The problem had been resolved and I'd received another reprieve from a death sentence. I was released the next day with a little bottle of pills in my hand and told to take one and one-half pills at an interval I can't recall. They were called quinidine, a derivative of quinine, and it was a cutting-edge medication of the time used to help regulate the heart.

I swore to myself I would be hyper-compliant when it came to taking those pills, that they would never be out of my pocket, and I would never go anywhere without them. And I did.

And now the real adventure was about to begin.

47

I kept the promise I'd made to myself about being hyper-compliant with taking the quinidine. My friends and I took a trip to Central Park, and I remember going out of my way to find water so I could take my pills as prescribed. That's the only activity I really remember of those few days. It was the night of April 25th. I vividly remember that the last thing I did was take my one and a half quinidine pills just before going to sleep. I was very excited. The next day was my seventeenth birthday, the one I almost didn't make. Little did I know it would also be the one I almost wouldn't live through.

48

When I first woke that next morning, I realized I had slept much longer than usual. But I couldn't get up. I felt groggy and foggy-headed and realized that something was wrong. All the alarms in my head went off at once. *Something is wrong.* I tried to take my pulse, something I had been doing obsessively since my release from LIJ, and I couldn't quite get it. So, I tried to get up and go to my mother who was home that day.

I tried to walk, and started towards the door of my bedroom, but it was as if I was drunk; I could barely walk or keep my balance. I looked at the clock and saw it was time to take my one and one-half quinidine again. I stumbled to the bottle, which was on my desk, opened it, and poured out one pill and the remaining half from the night before. There they sat, in the palm of my right hand, and all of my being, every fiber, *everything* in me, *screamed, Do Not Take Them!* When my body tells me something, I always listen, so I put the pills back in the bottle, put the cap on and placed them on the desk again. It's a good thing I did.

My mother must have heard me stir as she was coming towards my room, while I was trying to get out of it. "Good morning sleepy-head!" my mother brightly called before I was in view. I'm a night-owl by nature and it is common for me to stay up late and wake up late. But this was much later than normal, and my mother, as she later told me, thought I was just sleeping-in because it was my birthday.

I was almost at the door, in view of my mother who was waiting for me in the hall. I continued towards her and walked straight into the door jamb, just missing my face. Mom started laughing, thinking I was still not quite fully awake yet. She went to hug me and as she did, I just about collapsed in her arms. Her alarm bells rang. She walked me down the very short hall to the living room and the nearest chair in the house. I collapsed into it. My mother assessed me as a nurse, but with the urgency of a parent. I can still see her face and the combination of shock and concern it displayed.

Of course, she went right to my pulse. After she tried the first time, her face registered incredulity, and she took it again. Same result. She looked horrified. Forty-four, she told me. She called the doctor and explained the situation to him. When she hung the phone up she told me he'd said I was having a severe reaction to the quinidine. This happens to one in 10,000 patients. Surprise! Happy Birthday!

No, there would be no ambulance, no taking me by car back to the hospital. I was too fragile, it had been explained, and any kind of activity could push me over the edge. Lay me down, keep me in bed, and if I was stronger in the morning, bring me in then.

So, with my mother's help, we walked me back to my bed

where I laid down facing straight up. She took my pulse again. It was somewhere in the thirties. Any lower and, well, you know. Mom's emotions started to hit her just as something else started to hit me. Mom just started to cry, a lot, and while she was doing so, every fiber in my being was telling me, *This is it, Steven. This is the big one.* With every passing second, that message was getting stronger and stronger and louder and louder. *It's time to do battle, time to armor-up.* And while that message was being sent to me from I don't know where, I patted my mother on the back telling her everything was okay. *But it was time to do battle.* I had no time to waste consoling my mother. I needed everything I had to confront whatever it was that was coming. But here's what I *knew*: If I didn't get my mother out of there so I could concentrate, so *I could do battle*, I wasn't going to get out of that room alive.

Yes, I believe in miracles; not in the sense that most who believe in them do, but I believe in them nonetheless. And what followed will forever in my mind count as one of the true miracles of my life, because without it I don't believe I'd be here writing this. I don't remember my exact words, but I asked my mother to leave the room. One sentence. No arguing, no "I want to stay." She just said, "All right," kissed my forehead, got up, left the room and went into the backyard. It was almost as if she had become a robot under someone else's remote control. To this day I have trouble believing what I saw with my own eyes, but it happened and short of saying it was a miracle I have no other explanation for my mother, Momma Bear, leaving the room at that moment so quickly and with no protestations of any kind. It hadn't ever happened before, and it never happened again.

Like I said: A miracle. A miracle that saved my life.

49

I t didn't take long. Literally, within 30 seconds to a minute of my mother leaving my room, it hit me, and I mean, *it hit me.* I was lying on my back, thinking, wondering, and feeling apprehensive, to say the least. I knew something was coming, but I didn't know exactly what it was or in what form it would take when I got my answer. Like I said, it hit me, and it hit me suddenly. ***BAM!*** It felt like someone with perfect aim had swung a sledgehammer at my chest. It made me jump. It was unbelievably painful, unbelievably sudden. That was a big part of it; the suddenness. Then there was another blow, but not as strong. A couple more, each less of a blow until it just started to hurt; a constant hurt. A lot of pain. I clutched my chest, moaning and twisting right and left.

Shit, Steven, I said to myself, *how are you going to get out of this one?*

And then it started. I was lying there in pain, so much pain, and then, I swear, I heard the sound of something similar to a large, old light switch. *Click.* The most amazing things happened at that click. First, the pain went away, just dissipated like a puff of smoke. Poof. Gone. And then the show really began. At the same moment the pain disappeared, and exactly at the same instant of my hearing that *click*, I separated from my body. It was almost like in a cartoon when a character is pulling on something and then it lets go and goes *boing*. Well, that's as close as I can describe it, and, it's pretty close. It was as if my soul had to be pulled from me. Next thing I knew, I was looking down at myself, face to face. I relaxed. My hands dropped to my sides, and I'm pretty sure that was when my heart stopped as well.

Now, this is the really interesting part, at least it is to me. I never lost consciousness, not for a moment. I possessed two sets of vision and two consciousnesses and all were connected to at least some extent throughout the entire event. The part of me that was in the bed saw everything up to a point that my soul saw. And I truly believe it was my soul, that part of me that was leaving my body and making its slow ascent towards the ceiling. The part of me that was on the bed clearly saw the ceiling, but, at the same time, I also saw what my soul saw. So, while bed-me was looking at the ceiling, soul-me was looking down at my body, and I could see me from that perspective. It was incredible and oddly beautiful and very serene. The thing to remember is now I had two separate minds and two sets of vision and two separate lines of *thought*. Yeah, it confuses me, too. But I did not feel any pain, and for every inch my soul climbed, the most beautiful and calming peace enveloped both of me. *So, this is death. It's beautiful. Okay, it's fine—let's go*, I thought to myself on the bed. At that point the me on the bed wanted to die. No more battles, no more fighting, no more waiting for the other shoe to drop–just peace and bliss.

The me floating above me was having a different experience, however. The two experiences were identical until I reached my ceiling, whereupon the ceiling just dissolved away, allowing me to float through it. I could still see me on the bed. I watched and heard as the me on the bed said, *Oh wow.* I looked behind me and saw my mother in the backyard, next to our three-foot-high chain-link fence, talking to our neighbor, and then I looked up as I became enveloped by the blackest black I had ever seen. Below, I could no longer see me, but I knew I was still smiling, staring at the ceiling.

At first, I just kept floating and floating up. But there was more. Like I said, I was in the blackest black I had ever seen. Imagine this: Someone digs a hole 20 feet below the ground and puts a cement box, totally black inside and out, into that hole. Then you are put into that box, and the black cement lid is put on top of it, and then the hole is filled. *That* wouldn't be black enough to experience the black I was in.

But when I looked up and to the right there was a grayish light, the most beautiful light I had ever seen. This light was also the brightest light I had ever seen, the exact opposite of the black that consumed me, but it was grayish because I was far from it. Unbelievably far away. Unbelievably bright, yet it illuminated nothing but itself. If there was supposed to be a tunnel, I didn't see it. For me, and this may only apply to me, the "tunnel" is the shaft light makes when it pierces the dark. But I didn't see a tunnel. I did, however, see that light! All I wanted to do was get to that light, and while I was still ascending, that feeling of extreme peace and serenity was as tightly wrapped around me as the black that encased me. *Yes! Yes! This is fantastic! Yes, I'm coming!* It was at that moment I became part of All Knowledge. Everything. I knew the answer to absolutely everything. I understood every mystery of the Universe. I understood that there was no such thing as time, that it didn't matter if I had died when I was seven, or now at seventeen or if I was seventy! It was all the same! I couldn't wait to reach that light—that light that appeared to be *The Promise of Everything*.

Then something new started to happen. It all started to change. My ascension started to slow down. Instinctively, I knew that wasn't good. I was too far from the light. That was the point the me on the bed didn't go beyond, didn't get to see or experience. The me on the bed continued to be bathed in bliss and couldn't wait to die.

The light! I have to get to the light! I can't slow down now! But I did, and as I did, it became the coldest cold, down to your marrow cold, colder than anything that could ever be on earth cold. It was as cold as it was black. The slower my ascension, the colder it became.

I started to become aware that I wasn't alone. Far from it. It was crowded! My ascension stopped in an extraordinarily dense crowd. Now here is the strange thing. I couldn't see, in the conventional sense. The only thing I could "see" was the black and the light, and nothing else. But yet, I could somehow "see." Maybe a better word is *sense*, but not in any way that I could possibly describe here, that there *was* a crowd, a crowd as tightly packed as a Japanese commuter train. And everyone was cold, shivering, miserable and—I'm not kidding—gnashing their teeth. This had to be hell. After all, the Greek translation of the word *hell*, I've been told, is "absence of light." *NO! I can't be stuck here! I just wanted to get to the light! So, is this what hell is; stuck in a packed crowd of miserable souls, in the dark and cold, desperate to get to the light, a light that oddly gave no illumination, no warmth, that can't be reached, but is always there to tease you and show you what you could've had? Is that it? Is that what Hell is? Is this Hell? Where am I?*

By that time my soul was in a panic. That place was horrible beyond anything I'd ever encountered, beyond anything possible to experience in life. And then I felt it: a parting of the crowd. It wasn't unlike the way it feels when a cop moves through a crowd, a crowd so dense that others can't move, but that somehow a cop can push through. And as he does, the whole crowd can feel the parting, the wake, as it were, as the cop advances. Well, that's what it felt like. He, and I say *he* because of the timbre of his voice, came up behind my right shoulder, which was odd, as I no longer had a body, and put his hand on me, again odd. And I swear to this–this is the only way I can describe it: *in a voice I never heard before but that I recognized*, he said, "No, go back, you're not ready yet." Those were the exact words, contraction and all. I will never forget those words or how they sounded.

Okay, how do I get back? You will never be able to convince me that I didn't have help. The me on the bed, the blissfully happy me, the dunderhead who, up to that point, was unaware of all of this, somehow got the message. When bed-me understood, I said, out loud, "*Oh shit.*" I think at some level bed me did see that part of the event, but in a very distant way. I was disappointed. I didn't want to come back. My arms were still at my sides and some time had passed since the experience started. How long? I don't know. It could have been 30 seconds, it could have been 90, it could have been a minute or two. I have no way of knowing, but I got the message that somehow I was supposed to re-start my heart.

What gave me this idea, I will never know, but I am content to call it Divine Inspiration. For no reason that I can attribute to myself, and with what had to be the last possible thing I'd be able to do, I abruptly flung my arms with everything I had left across my chest.

Thump.

Oh my God, did that hurt! My blood was now in stasis, that is, my blood was no longer moving; just pooling in my veins and arteries. That first heartbeat jolted every single cell in my body, literally, as the blood was forced to move again.

Thump. More pain, but less, and less still with every beat. It was beating, but very slowly, and with no discernible rhythm. With each beat of my heart, my soul descended a small amount. It wasn't descending smoothly, only with each beat. I broke out of the darkness exactly where I had entered it, just above my roof. I saw my mother again, who was still talking to my neighbor. My ceiling dissolved, and I saw myself on the bed. Here's that confusing part again: the part of me that was on the bed still saw the ceiling, but my soul was again looking down on me.

Thump. Thump. Thump. Each beat acting like a ratchet, pulling me back down to earth, one click at a time, like a crew pulling on the ropes of a blimp hand-over-hand to bring it to its mooring. Finally, I was face-to-face again. I could feel my soul re-entering my body, and then I heard it. *Click*. Loud and clear, *Click*. Once again, I was body and soul. Whole.

At that moment, all the knowledge, everything I heard and experienced, was transferred to my tiny human brain. For a few seconds I struggled to retain it all, but it too, like a puff of smoke in a hurricane, just evaporated. Humans just can't understand, comprehend, nor retain that information. We're not meant to. It's too big for us. *It's not meant for us.* All that I kept was the experience itself, every aspect of it, and what I realized earlier about time, although the deep understanding I had of it disappeared, too. But I knew something else. I wasn't going to die, no matter how sick the pills had made me, no matter how unstable my heart had become, no matter how frightened my mother was, or what my doctors thought. *This was not my time to die. I'd actually been told.* As it would become clearly apparent during the next two days, I was the only one who knew or thought this. But right then, I was safe, comforted by the knowledge and experience I'd just been blessed with. I let out a huge sigh, let go of everything and just sagged into myself, exhausted from my journey.

50

A lot of this would have been hard for even me to believe if I didn't have proof of certain aspects of it. First, the book *On Death and Dying* by Elisabeth Kübler-Ross came out about six months *after* my birthday. I had never before heard of an out of body or near-death experience, as it is commonly called today. I had never heard about *The Light* or tunnels or any of it. When I finally went back to school and told several friends what had happened they all looked at me as if I were nuts. Only my closest friends believed me, or at least acted as if they believed me. I quickly got the hint and stopped telling others about what I had heard and seen. Several of them came back to me after *On Death and Dying* had been published and, after they had read it, told me they now believed me.

But my mother turned out to be the one that confirmed, for both of us, that I had indeed had experienced a NDE. Sometime after I had returned from my journey, my mother had come back to my room to check on me. For some reason, I didn't want to tell her everything, but I needed to know certain things for myself. I asked her if she had just been in the backyard. Yes. Were you standing by the fence talking to Mr. Lewis? Yes. Were you standing a little sideways to the fence, towards the house and was Mr. Lewis standing almost perpendicular to the fence? Yes. Was he wearing blue and green madras shorts and a white polo shirt? Yes. Was he wearing socks and sandals? Yes. Was he holding a pair of hedge clippers in his hands? Yes! Yes! Yes! My mother was astounded and understood immediately what all of that meant. She grabbed hold of me and started to cry, except this time she was crying for joy. You see, we both knew something. We both knew it was impossible for me to have seen my mother and Mr. Lewis from my room. It was physically impossible unless the window was open, and I was hanging out of it as far as I could. But even if I had done that, bushes and trees still would have blocked the view. Completely. That was all the conformation either of us needed. Not too long after the NDE, and after that entire event had run its course, I told my mother the whole story. She didn't have a single doubt about any of it.

I haven't told that story many times in my life. It is too special. I was afraid that if I told it too often it would both cheapen and make it change from the telling. I always knew I would write about it someday, as I am now, and I wanted the story in all its detail to be as pristine as possible for when I did. Fortunately, the story did stay true and I'm relieved that I have been able to convey it here accurately. It's almost as if a small burden has just been lifted. Last time I told this account some years ago to someone who was very close to me, he, very smugly and in a condensing tone, told me he didn't believe me. "Are you calling me a liar?" I asked. "No, I just don't believe you," he replied. I didn't see the difference. He went on to say that pilots and astronauts who are put in centrifuges for G-force training, and who sometimes black-out from the experience, often report that they see a light before they lose consciousness. Did they see their mother in the backyard and describe it perfectly, or did they see the control room where they were, or *anything*? No, just a light. But he still didn't believe me. So, I stopped telling the story. Until now.

When *On Death and Dying* came out, it became a media sensation. I couldn't get my hands on it fast enough. When I did, I practically devoured it. Almost all the experiences detailed in that book were pretty much the same, all almost identical to mine but with one huge exception: none of them had been caught in the cold and darkness the way I had. All spoke of the bliss I first felt, and the light, but none of them had their bliss turn to terror.

Why the difference?

That question has haunted me ever since the event. I thought about it then and I still do. It was my seventeenth birthday, the day of my NDE. What could I have done to deserve Hell at such a young age? I hadn't murdered anyone, (that's still true!) hadn't committed adultery or even had sex yet, didn't steal anything, so what could I have done that brought me there?

I think I know the answer, and I've only reached it recently. In most of the accounts found in *On Death and Dying*, those events lasted a lot longer than mine did. And, forgive me for how I say this—I just don't have any other way of putting it— but they might have been *more dead* than I had been. I don't know, but that's my best guess. But when I play back what the voice that told me, *"No, go back, you're not ready yet,"* and I again hear its deep, soothing gentleness, a voice that sounded like it came from someone who was *smiling*, the only conclusion I can reach is that I just didn't belong there in the first place. That just happened to be where my soul was stopped to be told that and then to go back. This conclusion rings true and satisfies me, and because of that, I no longer worry about it as I used to.

But this entire event wasn't over. I was still in trouble and both my mother and I knew it. I still had to get through the night, and if I did, which I knew I would, I'd have to go back to the hospital the next day. No, it wasn't over. I was still engaged in battle, still had a fight in front of me. I looked over to where the pills were sitting on my desk, immensely grateful that I had listened to myself and not taken them. I would have to listen to myself again the following day, but I didn't know that yet. I was just happy that I had listened on my birthday. I knew I still had to fight, but at least I also knew that I was going to live, if I continued to fight and listen to myself.

I still have that bottle of pills, the one with the half-pill in it. The half-pill and the others, one of which had I taken with that half-pill, would have killed me. Killed me dead.

51

Next morning came and, as soon as I woke, my mother was on the phone with the doctor. My heart was beating, but it was extremely irregular. It was determined that I was strong enough to get to the hospital. With my mother's help I was able to get in her car. I was weak, as weak as a ninety-three-year-old woman without her walker. That was okay, because once I got to the hospital, I was put in a wheelchair and taken to the ICU. I may have been weak, but my spirits were still flying high from the NDE. Believe it or not, I did then, and I still do now, consider my seventeenth birthday to be the best birthday of my life. That NDE was the best gift I have ever been given.

That was how I was feeling as they wheeled me into my room at Manhasset Hospital, the closest hospital to my home. It was also the hospital where my doctor's office was and where my mother worked. On the right-hand wall of the hall just before my room was a cardiac monitor sitting on a cart. A bell went off in my head when I saw it. My room was bright and sunny, with lots of windows that faced north and looked down on Northern Boulevard. If I looked behind me, I could see a funeral home that was next to the hospital. How convenient, I thought. The irony of that made me smile. If memory serves me correctly, I was on the sixth floor. Mine was the only bed in the room, even though it seemed like it was large enough for another. There was a little cabinet next to the bed, a rolling tray table for eating that was set to the side at that time, and the obligatory privacy curtain hanging from its rails but pushed all the way to one side of the bed behind my left side. That was it. There was no phone or television.

I'd had a heart-block incident the previous day, it was explained. Call it an electrical heart attack, of sorts. My negative reaction to the drug had caused the electrical signal from my brain to my heart to be blocked, so my heart had decided it didn't have to beat any more. That is, until I told it to get back to work. Nonetheless, what all this meant was that I was fragile, and that the doctors, my mother, and now the entire family didn't know if I'd survive the day. Of course, I wasn't told *that* part, but I knew what they were thinking. It was all over their faces. Really, how could I not know? I mean, come on, they were afraid to even give me an *aspirin*, or anything else for that matter. I was told that I wasn't to have a TV or radio because they didn't want me to get excited in the least, which could provide that final push over the edge. Apparently, in order to live I was going to have to be bored to death.

After that event was all over, my mother told me how they feared I wouldn't make it through the night. By then my father and my brother Michael had both driven in from their respective dwellings in New Jersey. It was Michael who told me that the doctor had told him and my parents to "make arrangements" because he didn't think I'd make it through the night. Also, my mother had called my friend Joe's mother. Joe told me that when his mother told him I was in the hospital again he responded by asking how I was, and she had replied sadly, and this is a quote, "It's very bad. It doesn't look good."

While all of this was going on, one of the nurses had applied the leads to me with a strap that went around my chest that was wired to a cardiac monitor in the nurses' station. While the nurse was doing this, I asked her if I could have the monitor that was in the hall. I was told no, it wasn't necessary, that they were monitoring me at the nurses' station. I asked again and was again told no, only a little more firmly.

But this was *me* listening to me again. In the same way, and with the same force that my body told me not to take those pills, it was now demanding that I get that monitor moved into my room. *My life depended on it.* I don't know how I got those thoughts or where they came from or even *how* my life would depend on that monitor, but I got the message loud and clear. All I did know was that if I was being told my life depended on that monitor, then I was going to get it, *had* to get it, and that made it my job *to* get it. Period.

My doctor then came in to visit me and I told him I wanted the monitor from the hall and to be taught how to use it. He pretty much told me what the nurse had said just a little while before. Doctor, I want that monitor. No, you're being monitored. We went back and forth a few times and then I made my threat, one I had every intention of realizing if I didn't get my way. I looked him right in the eye and said, "Doctor, either you give me that monitor and teach me how to use it, or I will get up on this bed and jump up and down and scream." He looked shocked and took a step back, almost as if the force of my words had physically pushed him. He believed me, and it was a good thing he did, because I was a moment from making good on my threat, and for all intents and purposes, committing suicide in front of him. To my thinking, that was the only way I could get that monitor. And if my life depended on getting it and I couldn't, well then—I'd rather die on my own terms.

You cannot underestimate how much power the NDE had given me, especially those words, those unbelievably powerful words, *"No, go back, you're not ready yet."* I'm not saying this in a cocky way. I'm just stating what was, which is that I was now operating on a different plane, one that no one but me could possibly understand. I had my orders, as it were, and my protection. I had to operate based on my own instincts, what my body was telling me, and on the grace of whatever Divine Inspiration was telling me. The doctors, my family, *none of them*, had a clue as far as I was concerned. How could they? They hadn't seen what I had, hadn't heard what I had, and hadn't been promised what I had. I knew two things: I would die without that monitor and something told me that my threat would be enough, even though I would have carried it out if I didn't get what I needed.

Less than two minutes later that same nurse who told me no, wheeled the monitor, with its cart, to the right side of my bed and added the additional leads to my chest to hook me up to the machine.

Let me explain a little about cardiac monitors from the late sixties. They were gigantic, the size of the original microwave ovens. And for all that bulk, they had just a tiny, four-inch-in-diameter, green cathode-ray tube (CRT). That is where the little squiggly line that traced your heartbeat appeared. Today, they are the size of a notebook computer. Again, I got to hear a nurse mutter the word *brat* in my direction, but, honestly, I couldn't care less about what she thought. She, like all the others, didn't know and was, frankly, ignorant of the true situation. I really can't blame her when looking at it from her perspective. She showed me how to work it, (it was very simple, really) and she left in a huff that was meant for my benefit.

I turned to that screen and watched the terribly irregular trace of my heartbeat accompanied by the unsteady *beep* that went along with it. I started to stare at that screen, as I would do almost continuously for the next three days.

I had been given my weapon and Divine Inspiration was now telling me how to employ it. I was ready. Time to fight.

52

I stared at that screen as if my life depended on it because it did. I promptly understood why I needed it. My new battle, my *job*, was to *will* my heart to beat, and to beat *constantly and with more regularity*. Sounds strange, doesn't it? Well, you would understand as quickly as did I if you saw what I saw on that screen.

My new problem was arrhythmia, or an irregular heartbeat. Lots of people have irregular heartbeats, but mine was severe. Let me explain the difference. Instead of a heartbeat that went *Thump... Thump... Thump... Thump... Thump... Thump...* and so on, my heartbeat was so irregular that most of the time the monitor would register only one or two heartbeats per sweep, as long as it took for the line to go across the screen—about four or five seconds. It was common for no heartbeat to register per sweep, or for even two and a half sweeps, and several times, not just a couple, but maybe 20 times or so–I didn't have a beat for almost three and a half full screens! That'll get your attention. Imagine yourself looking at a monitor of your heartbeat where it's a literal flat line for even one sweep of the screen. Those times of three sweeps or more without a beat were long enough for the blood to start to go stasis, and then the next beat would always come as a little and slightly painful jolt, albeit a very welcome one.

On those occasions where it didn't beat for two or more screens, I was practically yelling at my heart to get back to work (in my head, of course). The rest of the time, I was just staring at that screen, or more precisely the line on the screen, *willing* it to beat more regularly, actively imagining a beat where there was none. *Come on. Come on–BEAT.* I did this for hours on end, almost all the time I was awake for the first two days. If I did sleep, I'd wake just to check—to make sure my heart wasn't falling down on the job. My sleep for the first couple of days was uneasy at best.

After a few days, it did get more regular, much to the surprise of everyone but me. Hell, everyone was shocked that I made it through that first night! By the second day I think my mother figured out that I wasn't going anywhere, and she calmed down to whatever extent she was capable of calming down under those circumstances.

All through that event my spirits were up. *Yeah, I had to fight.* My life wasn't just being given back to me complete with a magical cure. *No, I had to fight for it.* But that didn't matter because I knew what I knew, and that made me completely confident on what the outcome would be. Let's suppose I did die the next day or the day after that. I was also confident that if I did, well then, it *would've* been my time and therefore I had nothing to fear in that case, either. For the most part, I was happy for those days, fight or not.

Nowadays they call what I did bio feedback, but that concept wasn't around back then, at least not that I'd ever heard of. Nor had anyone else I knew, including my doctor. I really don't take credit for any of this. By that I mean the fact I knew I needed that monitor and understood the way I needed to employ it. Divine Inspiration is the only thing that explains this for me, and I'm happy with that conclusion. By the way, weeks after that event, during an office visit, my doctor told me that the only reason I was alive was because of me. My birthday blessing.

Toward the end of my stay in the ICU and before I was moved to a regular room, I had been given two things to help combat the boredom. My heart was beating more regularly by then, and although it was still very irregular, at least it had improved enough that I didn't feel the need to stare at the monitor the way I previously had. The first thing I was given was Hemingway's novel, *The Sun Also Rises,* along with a couple of sheets of paper and a pencil. It was a good story, but I wasn't able to finish it because it stayed in the ICU when I was moved. The paper was a different story, and, in a strange way, I used it as I had the monitor. I drew a picture of myself as I thought I'd look in the future, about the same age I am now. Those were the days of hippies and long hair, (1971) and I was a hippie and had long hair. Hippie or not, I'd never used drugs because I was always afraid of what they would do to my heart. At seventeen I promised myself I would always have long hair and be interested in music. I had an agency that booked local bands in local venues. In short, I didn't want to be what I thought of as, looking through my seventeen-year-old eyes, a sell-out.

I drew a picture of Future Me, in profile. I made a promise to myself that when I attained that age—50 or so I would look like my drawing. In the drawing I was bald, because I thought I'd be bald, but thankfully that never came true. I had an earring in my left ear, a gold hoop, and I was sporting a goatee. So, how did I do? Well, I tried to get the earring in my freshman year in college, but it wouldn't take and hurt so much I dropped the idea entirely. I've had facial hair of one sort or another for most of my teenage and adult life, so I was covered in that regard, (pardon the pun) and I have a goatee now. Then, a few years ago, I was looking at myself in the mirror and the promise I made to that seventeen-year-old-boy came rushing back to me. It hit me kind of hard. So, then and there I decided to start growing my hair to where it reached the bottom of my shoulder blades. My wife hated it. She hated even more the fact that I didn't care that she hated it. A lot of people didn't like it. But they didn't understand, even though I explained that something bigger was going on, something important. At least it was to me. I wore it long for a few years, and satisfied I had kept my promise, I cut it.

Why do I care so much about a promise I made decades ago? Because I equate that drawing with the cardiac monitor; it helped save my life. I would stare at that drawing, and just in the same way I was willing my heart to beat, here I was willing myself to grow old, something that many never thought would happen. But it did. When I went to my fortieth high school reunion, more than one person ran up to me yelling, "You're still alive!" Yeah, I am, and I believe that a good part of the reason that I'm still here is that drawing, that drawing that I framed and have hanging in my office, that drawing I made a promise to seventeen-year-old me.

And that's why, even if it's was only for a short while, I had long hair. I promised that little boy, and I don't give a darn what anyone thought of it. A promise is a promise.

53

I was moved to a room with two beds, one of which was already occupied. My new roommate was a man in his fifties, and I swear he was Archie Bunker's (from the seventies sitcom *All in The Family*) double—both in appearance and attitude. He took one look at his new hippie roommate and groaned out loud in displeasure, just as Archie would have. Let's just say he wasn't shy about letting his feelings be known. He was a nice enough man underneath it all, and he worked for the Postal Service.

Our beds were perpendicular to each other, his next to the window and mine next to the wall that had the door to the room. But to hell with not having the view; I had something much more valuable: I had a phone! A dull green, rotary phone! Oh, it was such a thing of beauty. After being alone in a room for four or five days, with almost no human contact, that phone represented a sort of freedom to me; it was as if the gates to my solitary confinement had just been flung open.

I was no longer on a monitor, but I wasn't allowed out of bed to walk. I was still being restricted in activity. I must have been allowed to use the bathroom, because I don't remember using a bedpan. But I believe if I'd had to use a bedpan in front of Archie, privacy curtain or not, I would have remembered it.

I couldn't wait to get to that phone, to be able to call my friends and let them know I was all right and to catch up on things. I have to say the responses were heart-warming and did wonders for my morale. And the phone rang at least as often as I used it to make calls.

My second day in that room did even more for my morale. Those were the days when hospitals held strict visiting hours, and they were pretty rigorous about maintaining the rules that governed them. There were two or three blocks of visiting hours a day, each set, I think, for two hours each. Visitors were restricted to 15 minutes during each visiting block. Only two people were allowed to visit at any one time, and in order to visit you had to go to the visitors' desk and get a pass. There were only two passes per patient. Honestly, I never understood rules like these. I think the less doctors know the stricter they are. I think it was a way to cover the fact that they *didn't know* how visitors would affect patients, but a rule like that made it appear as if they did. Look, I love doctors. I owe my life to them, but like anyone else, they aren't perfect. Although I have known several who would argue with you about that last point.

Well, apparently my friends felt the same way about those visitation rules, and they decided to make rules of their own. Two of my friends, both with the requisite passes, came to visit. Both had long hair, which, as you can imagine, just *thrilled* Archie. They were classmates and members of a band I managed, and they told me they had a surprise for me. The surprise was at that moment making its way up the fire stairs. It was a bunch of my classmates. A minute later, they all made their way to my room. All of them, male and female were hippies, and they and I were ecstatic to see one another. There were literally about 15 to 20 kids in our small room. We were laughing and crying and hugging; it was wonderful and something I really needed. I didn't know I needed it as badly as I did until they all showed up.

There was also a facet to that visit that was quite unexpected as well: a lot of them spoke to Archie and his family. His wife and very beautiful daughter, who was about the same age as me, were also there at the time. You could see the shock register on their faces, as hippie after hippie piled into the room. What must have been more surprising, at least to Archie and his wife, were that they were all respectful and basically nice kids. Many of them introduced themselves to him and his family. My friends asked him how he was doing, what was wrong with him, how soon it would it be till he went home, and they all wished him well. During all this the wife just looked bewildered, while the daughter seemed to enjoy the attention. She was a knockout and every guy noticed.

It was awesome. I don't know if I possess the vocabulary that could relate both how joyously happy this visit made me and what it meant to me then and even now. It was one of the times when I felt most loved in my life. I get a warm feeling whenever I think about it. The room was literally packed.

We all knew visiting time was over when we heard the screech of the nurse who discovered the situation. She started ordering everyone out of the room, pulling some by their arms and directing the rest with a waving hand. She was quite indignant about the whole thing, which was hysterical to us. The horror! The gross violation of the visiting hour rules! What's next? Visiting whenever you want? Really, her indignation was hilarious.

I know she said something about this breach of the sacred

rules to me when the room had been cleared, but whatever it was I didn't hear it. I don't think I would have cared if I did. I was flying. I was too happy, too filled with joy, at the gift my friends had just given me to hear a word she said.

And here is something that truly surprised me: Archie. Even though he had a lot to say afterwards about the length of my friends' hair and how they dressed, that mass visit somehow softened him. The edge, if not his entire attitude, had lessened. I think he respected that I had many people who cared about me as much as they did, and that they had all been concerned for him, too. Also, I think the madhouse we had for as many minutes that the visit lasted had somehow cheered him up, as well. I also sense it made him re-think what he thought of hippies, even if it was only by a degree or two.

When my mother came to visit later, I told her what had transpired, including the screeching nurse. She laughed and thought the whole thing was a riot, too.

I slept well that night.

54

I spent more than a week or so in the hospital that time around, and when I was released my heartbeat was far from regular. I think the hope was it would eventually even out on its own over some period of time. But truth be told, released or not, I was still in trouble.

Trouble or not, I'd moved into a new realm, a new place as to how I looked at the world and how I was going to deal with death. Make no mistake, death was still stalking me. I knew it and death knew it, and we continued to eye each other suspiciously. Part of my new strategy was to dare death and spit him in the eye and act like he wasn't there, even though I knew he was.

I'd started smoking cigarettes when I was thirteen, partially, as part of my denial of death, and then I started to smoke more. Soon I was up to three packs a day of Tareyton 100's. You can imagine how this went over with my mother, my doctor and my friends. I remember one beautiful spring day shortly after returning to school from the hospital, when, during a break from class, I lit one up while sitting on the concrete stairs that were to the side of the main entrance of the school. My friend, David, saw this from about 40 feet away and came running at me as if to push me out of the way of an oncoming train. With a final yell he launched at me, landed on me, and we both tumbled down the stairs, the *concrete* stairs, about two or three steps to the ground, which was also concrete. We were a tangled mess when we landed. I was consumed with laughter as I pointed out to him that making us both fall down concrete steps might be more immediately harmful to us than me lighting up a single cigarette. David didn't think anything about it was funny. Well, maybe a little bit, but he didn't want me to smoke. But in spite of his and others' efforts to get me to stop, I continued to smoke anyway. They didn't understand. I was busy spitting in the eye of death.

Then there was Joe to deal with. He was upset with me that I hadn't told him I had a year to live. I explained how I didn't want to see that look in his eye that I knew would at some point, or points, show up. The pity, the sadness. I explained how that would have sapped my strength. He understood, but only to a point. He made me promise he would be in the loop if anything similar happened in the future.

When Joe did visit me in the hospital, he gave me a card. It was a condolence card and he'd written RIP, "Rest in Peace," on the front. That was Joe and I, and our relationship, to a tee. I, of course, found the card to be very funny, while it deeply offended my mother. She got over it. Joe told me when he went to buy the card the lady in the shop was quite confused as to why he was buying a condolence card for someone who hadn't died yet. How I wish I could have seen that exchange!

I was in my new realm and busy taking command of my new territory. I was always a worker, but now I went berserk. I worked whenever and wherever I could. On weekends I was working at a very high-end restaurant as a busboy, making an average of $90 to $110 over two nights. That was a lot of money back then, since you could rent a nice two-bedroom apartment for about $150 a month. During weekend days I was working on a three-acre estate with a pool as their gardener/handyman.

There was something that told me that physical labor would be good for my heart, and, as always, I listened when "something" told me, well, *something*. And besides, I was busy chasing life with a hammer. I was going to be rich and famous someday, and people were going to remember my name, and that ultimately would have me beating death at its own game. Or so I thought back then. Bottom line? Death was not going to erase Steven G. Taibbi.

Be that as it may, as the months went on and my arrhythmia didn't improve, I had several frank conversations with my doctor. He wanted me to get a pacemaker. I didn't. He said it was essential. I didn't care. No, I don't want one.

Why was I adverse to a pacemaker? I can't really tell you other than I didn't want one. Maybe I just didn't want another surgery. Maybe I didn't want something that would have me in the hospital for maintenance on a regular basis. I just know I didn't want it. My mother wanted me to get it, but I firmly told her no. I was still a minor when this debate was going on. My mother might have been able to overrule me, but she didn't. In some odd way, my mother and I were always in tune with each other, and after I told her no, she dropped the subject.

Then the doctor told my mother and me that he thought my time on this earth was limited. In his estimation, he didn't think I'd make thirty. Hell, he wasn't sure I'd get past my mid-twenties. Maybe so. But I had my hammer and I was busy chasing life with it. That was part of my new realm. I was going to be too busy to die. I was staring death right in the eye and challenging him to come and get me. *Screw you, death. I've changed. I'm not afraid of you.* My birthday gift had taught me invaluable lessons; lessons most don't learn until they near the end of their lives. But I knew it was part of my gift and that lesson was this: No matter what, no matter when, I was going to die. It's like the night, it's coming, and you have no way to stop it. None of us know how long our "day" will be. Some don't get past dawn, some almost make it to the next sunrise. Doesn't matter. It is what it is.

My other great gift was that I'd learned to embrace my death; accept it fully. Now, that may sound funny coming from a guy who was busy spitting death in the eye, but if you think about it, it makes sense. Death had been actively stalking me since the day I was born. I had to go through things none of my classmates had to endure. By spitting in death's eye, I was telling death, "I don't fear you. You won't have me cowering in a closet. I'm going to live while I have my life and I'm going to die on my own terms." But that was only possible because I'd made peace with the fact I was going to die. Have you, dear reader? Embrace your death and you will have the freedom to live.

There is a passage in the Bible that I think is misunderstood by almost everyone, or at least they don't get its "second" meaning. Most only get half its meaning and miss the half that is just as important. John, 12:25 says, "He who loves his life shall lose it, and he who hates his life in this world will keep it for eternal life." It's the first half of this passage that I think has two meanings, at least it does for me. "*He who loves his life shall lose it*" I interpret to mean if you love your life so much, if you're so afraid of dying, well, then you will never *live*. You will never have the courage to take risks, be out on your own, to dare to dream and make those dreams a reality, strike your own path, to *LIVE*, fully, to be wonderfully alive, if you are afraid, *terrified*, of your own death. Like I said before, *Death is like the night – it's coming.*

This was my new realm; my new understanding, my new *strategy*. My wife and my current doctors all have instructions that if it is at all possible, I want to be awake when I die. I want to be there when it happens. I want to experience it fully. I want to be able to pray as it happens and experience the transition. I want to meet the Voice and thank him. I want to be there, fully awake and grateful for all the special gifts I've been given. After all, this is the one and only event that I'm truly waiting my whole life for. I don't want to miss it.

In the meantime, I have my hammer and I'm busy chasing life with it.

55

So, I'd set my agenda for myself. I was going to work hard, become rich, only do things I wanted to do and live my life.

I kept my promise to Joe, and about a week after the doctor told me about not getting through twenty, I told him. We were on one of our long walks, something that we did often, and I remember stopping and telling him I had something to say. I don't remember the exact words, but I do remember the gist. I told him I really didn't want to tell him, but that I had said I would, so I was. I remember admonishing him that we wouldn't talk about it, that it was between us, and that I never wanted to see a look of pity or sadness cross his face when it came to this situation. We both kept our promises and Joe, outside of my mother and doctor, was the only other person to know.

I graduated high school, went to Quinnipiac College in Connecticut for almost a year, but was thrown out just before finals because my father didn't pay the tuition, which the divorce decree required. Déjà-vu all over again. That meant my second semester was a waste because it wouldn't count. That started a battle between my mother and father that ultimately set a precedent in the New York State Supreme Court. I went to work in a factory, full time, for a year and a half to help get the money to release my transcripts.

My mother, through great sacrifice, came up with the money, got my transcripts released, and I attended New York Institute of Technology in Brookville Long Island, which was commuting distance from my mother's house where I was living. After Quinnipiac, all—and I mean *all*— college expenses were up to me. I carried 21 credits a semester and worked three jobs, seven days a week, while also maintaining two internships.

I qualified for a small—and I mean *small*—grant every semester, which didn't even cover the cost of textbooks. I held many jobs while at Tech. During summer vacations, spring and winter breaks, I went back to the factory fulltime, even if it was just for two weeks. I detailed cars, wrote six car repair manuals and became an assistant manager/manager at a store chain. I also became a mechanic because my MGB—a little red British sports car—had forced me into it. I sold that car, which I dearly loved, in spite of its propensity for leaking oil and breaking one way or another every two weeks to help with my second semester tuition at Tech. I continued as a mechanic after that. I also flipped cars. I would buy a car for a hundred bucks or so, tune it and make any necessary repairs at the shop where I worked, clean it up and sell it for two hundred or so. Every little bit helped. My senior year, I had six cars and flipped five of them.

I barely ate. I would go days, sometimes four in a row, where all I had time for, and all I could afford, were candy bars, two or three of them a day. My mother would feed me if I was home, but I was always working or going to school, and as such, she didn't get much of a chance to help me in that way.

I paid for school, my books, transportation, car insurance, my own phone, worked like a dog, and—surprise, surprise—I thought it was great. I enjoyed school. I love to learn, and I was learning both at school and my jobs. I felt amazingly productive. I love that feeling as much as I love learning. Also, I had developed strategies for school that worked like a charm. One, I never missed a class. Why would I? That would be like throwing my own money out the window, and the teachers appreciated that I showed up for every session. They took it as a sign of commitment, which it was. Second, what textbooks I did buy, I bought used. And I saved even more money by not buying all the required books the courses asked for because of something else I learned. For 90 percent of the teachers, the books didn't matter. No, what mattered to them was what came out of their mouths during class. That was a life-saving revelation to me; one that cut my homework time drastically. What I did instead was develop my own sort of short-hand and, with it, I would take copious notes. It wasn't hard to determine when a prof was passionate about an element of a subject, or even if it was just that he thought a particular point was important. At these times, I would concentrate even harder on the exact words he or she would use.

When it came time for a test, I'd study the night and morning before, not with a textbook, but with my notebooks. Worked every time. Well, almost. To most of the professors, what they said was more important than what we were told to read. All I had to do was remember what they said in class. I always passed with flying colors. The best part was that I still learned the courses—just not from the textbooks. Truth be told, lots of my professors had insights that were worthwhile, insights the books often lacked. This strategy, unfortunately, didn't work for economics. I never understood why someone in a BFA program had to study economics. I struggled with it. *Struggled!* For me, the textbook was next to impossible to read, let alone understand, and I got a C+ when all was said and done. At graduation I missed Magnum Cum Laude by a tenth of a point because of that one course. I felt as if I had been robbed. I still do. I worked hard in college. I studied hard, attended all my classes, worked three jobs and two internships every semester, and yet I missed that honor because I was forced to take a course that had nothing to do with my degree. It was taught by a stubborn old man who couldn't communicate and used a textbook that might as well have been written in another language.

Regardless, I had put myself through college. Yeah, I had college loans and would pay them off in full, but I *owned* my education in a way that few others I'd gone to school with could claim. I dare say, I got more out of my education than most of my classmates did because I paid for it myself and my strategy required that I attend classes and pay attention. While most of my classmates came to school in cars paid for by their parents to attend classes also paid for by their parents, I could clearly see the difference between them and myself. Their attitude towards school was almost cavalier. To so many of them, school was a place to party and hang out. It wasn't worth as much to them as it was to me because it was being *given* to them. For me, however, school was precious and expensive, and I needed to get every penny's worth out of it. I will always be grateful I had to pay my own way through school. It did me a lot of good and I still feel the pride of accomplishment and continue to reap the benefits of everything I learned, both in and out of class.

All through this time, my arrhythmia became slightly better, but only slightly. As far as my prognosis was concerned, nothing had changed. And even though my mother and Joe didn't discuss this with me, it was always there, sometimes deep in the background, sometimes right in my face. I was dating a nurse who couldn't rest her head on my chest because of how greatly the rhythm of my heart disturbed her. A couple of times it disturbed her so much that she not only removed her head from my chest, she got up and left the room entirely. Also, during this time (and later) there were nights when my heart was incredibly irregular, the pounding so strong that I wasn't sure I'd make it through the night. On those occasions, I would say the Lord's Prayer, and force myself to sleep knowing that wherever I was when I awakened would be where I was supposed to be and that would be okay.

When I did wake after such a night, I'd say a prayer of thanks and then, once again, pick up my hammer and start the chase anew.

56

I started my freelance television production business two weeks before I graduated college. My first client was AT&T before it was broken-up by the government. I stayed with them afterwards, too. That's where I cut my teeth on television production and moved on from there. My next corporate client was Merrill Lynch. Pretty soon I had a good business going. I was working on national commercials and television shows and did a lot of work in this new thing called cable TV. At one point, I was working on the top-three-rated cable shows at the same time.

I had other side business, as well, and having the time of my life. I wasn't rich, but I was doing well. One of my dreams always seemed to elude me, however, and that was to become a pilot. With a medical history such as mine, I'd be required to have my doctor sign off on my pilot's license, as well as pass the separate FAA medical. Without that signature it was hopeless, and my doctor had made it clear he didn't want me to fly. Some years ago, I'd even tried the military, but after they heard of my medical history I was refused by the Air Force, the Navy and the Army (helicopters). My last resort was the Coast Guard. The gentleman I spoke with over the phone at the Guard listened to me patiently and empathically. He heard my deep desire to become a pilot. Finally, in a very soothing and fatherly tone he said something like this: "Son, I know you want to be a pilot and you want to serve, but with your medical history it just won't be possible for you, not with any of the branches. Just see what you can do to become a private pilot. You have no idea how sorry I am to have to tell you this."

He mollified me to a small extent, and I thanked him sincerely. Every time I think of him I'm grateful for how kindly he dealt with me. But when we got off the phone, I cried. I cried for myself and how once again my heart was going to deny me something I wanted badly, something most others who, if it had been their dream, would have been able to pursue. I always tried to look past the limitations of my heart condition, but I had wanted to be a pilot since my father used to throw Neiani and me through the air and onto his bed on some Sunday mornings. I loved the thrill of soaring through the air. I looked forward to those Sundays. *Sky King* and *The Whirlybirds* were my favorite childhood TV shows. I wanted to fly! And, as mentioned earlier, when I was in the hospital as a child, I would routinely escape whatever the current horrible reality was by soaring away from it all by riding on the back of my imaginary seagull. But, no matter how badly I wanted to fly, that door had now been firmly shut in my face, courtesy of my heart. I rarely felt sorry for myself, and this happened during the time when my doctor thought I had a limited life span, which I didn't mention to any of the recruiters, but none of that mattered to me. During the entire time of this prognosis, I was in full-blown bully-my-heart mode. I just couldn't accept that I wasn't able to bully my heart, or my doctor, to do this one thing. But that conversation with the kind Coast Guard recruiter had for some reason done me in. This is the only time I can think of when I cried because of the limitations my heart imposed on me.

But I *was* bullying my heart. Every day at some point I'd bully my heart in one way or the other. Ever since the doctor had given me the news about my limited lifespan, a huge part of me believed I could—I *would*—beat this thing, just as I had that last stay in the hospital. I bullied my heart there and I bullied my heart then. Mind over matter. Mind over heart. Mind over life. Part of my strategy was to do the exact opposite of what my doctor told me. That was one of the reasons I smoked that much, even though I'd given that up on my own—three packs a day, cold turkey—my freshman year.

One day, work took me to Bedminster, in the beautiful countryside of New Jersey. In what, for me, was a "meant-to-be moment," I had decided to take my break outside. It was a magnificent spring day. I was joined by a colleague named Shawn, someone I'd gone to NYIT with. In my whole career, this was the one and only time we worked together. As I said, a meant-to-be moment. When Shawn joined me, he saw I was staring into the sky. He lifted his gaze to see what I was so enthralled with. Sailplanes, also known as *gliders*, were doing graceful pirouettes in the air. They seemed as elegant as any seagull ever was. It was beautiful. My heart ached with the desire to be up there with them.

Shawn said the gliders were from Somerset Airport, just a mile or two away. Then he told me that it was where *he* learned to fly gliders and that he had been at that airport on a regular basis, but not as much lately. I turned to him, I'm sure with visible disappointment etched on my face and said I wished that I could do that. He said I could. I explained that because of my heart condition I wouldn't be able to pass the medical. He turned to look at me squarely and asked if I had a driver's license. Of course, I did. How do you think I got here? Well then, he said, you can fly gliders. There is no medical needed to become a sailplane pilot. All you need is to be healthy enough to drive.

The joy that burst within me at that moment was indescribable. I was practically jumping up and down! Shawn then gave me the address of the airport and the name of his instructor, Charlton Rehr. Shawn told me that she was the best soaring instructor anywhere near here and gave me her number. Once again, I did the exact opposite of what my doctor wanted and started my lessons to become a pilot two weeks later. And besides, it had seemed to me that my arrhythmia was getting better. But even if I didn't think that, I would have started the lessons anyway.

Something else, other than my heart, was going on, too. It had started when I was five and just continued to grow worse and worse with each passing year. There was, and I *knew* this to be true, something deeply, fundamentally wrong with me. I couldn't tell you what it was outright, but I knew it was something, nevertheless. The best way I can describe it is I knew I was *bad*. All through the hospital stays when I was five and six, I was told to be a good boy. *Be a good boy!* I thought I had been, I certainly tried, but, somehow, I thought I was never good enough. I still blamed myself and my illness for breaking up the family, and there had to be a reason why I went through all that I went through when no one else in my family or school had to go through the same thing. I just wasn't *good enough*. I *deserved* to be sick and unpopular. I deserved to suffer. I just knew that inside, somehow and for some reason, I was bad and would always be punished for it, then to forever. My being a good boy would never make any difference, because good boy or not, I wasn't good enough in the first place.

This led to a lot of self-sabotaging behavior. I ruined relationships that could have been magical. It was just that I knew, eventually, they'd see this horrible whatever it was thing in me that made me so bad, and they'd leave in disgust anyway. My business could have been much bigger if I hadn't kept self-sabotaging it. Maybe the worst thing of all was that silence terrified me. I mean absolutely *terrified* me. It still does, although to a lesser degree lately. Whether I was in a group or just with another person, I couldn't countenance silence. I would talk. It was as if that silence would allow something, some monster, out of the gate for the others to see, or worse let something in that could attack me. So, I would talk. I was always afraid I'd get rejected again. I'd been rejected so often, I was always nervous, always afraid of being rejected again. Also, I was terrified another shoe was going to drop. What that "shoe" would portend, or what that "shoe" would be, I had no idea, but I was terrified of it. many had dropped already.

Underneath that layer of terror was another layer, one that was even harder to bear than the terror: shame. I was ashamed from all those times in the hospital where I was treated like a piece of meat or stripped of my clothes in front of male and female medical students, or forcefully given an enema in front of a group of female nuns. I was always aware that I was a disappointment to my father and that my grandfather couldn't stand my company. I was ashamed because I was that person everyone thought they could pick on and bully, always the one to be rejected and humiliated in front of a group. Ashamed because I was the one that was bullied and made fun of, always the butt of the joke that had the whole class laughing *at* me. They knew. All of them knew that I was no good, that I was bad, that there was some secret mark on me that they could clearly see that told them to shun me, to belittle me, *because I was no good.* There was just something wrong with me, and because of that I deserved everything I got. I was ashamed that I was bad.

Underneath it all, in all the years of my life since I was five, I have lived with this terror. And, *terror* is not an exaggeration. No matter what I'm doing or where I am, it was and is always there at some level and some intensity. And just like the caboose at the end of the train, my terror pulled my shame along with it wherever I went. I have to tell you, Dear Reader, I'm ashamed for admitting this to you now.

Finally, though, I had found the one place where I could go where this terror and shame had the least hold on me—on the back of my seagull. Only this time it was real, and it was while I was at 5,000 feet in a single-place glider, soaring and executing exquisite pirouettes in the skies over Bedminster, New Jersey.

57

So, I had become a real pilot with a real pilot's license, rated to fly gliders and spending two to three, sometimes four days at the airport a week. I bought a used pop-up camper and put it behind a hangar owned by Al, the FAA rep at our airport who administered my *practical*, or final flying exam. Upon landing, Al had clapped his hand on my right shoulder as he said, "Congratulations! You're now a pilot!" I was so nervous from the test it took a few moments for me to register exactly what those words, words I can still hear and will never forget, meant.

I ran an extension cord from Al's hangar to the trailer for my electricity. While I was there, life was as perfect for me as it could get. I was camping in, for all intents and purposes, a canvas tent set above the ground, with a fiberglass roof. I always slept like a baby there and, if I was quiet, I could watch the deer graze just yards away. Best of all, when I woke, I woke at my airport where I was a short walk from renting a glider and going soaring.

During this time, I decided I had to come clean with my

doctor, so on a visit I told him I had become a pilot. He stood there, staring at me while his face changed from color to color. He was mad! But he kept his calm as well as he could and with a wagging, pointed finger inches from my face, said, "Okay, just no acrobatics!" What I didn't tell him was that as part of the curriculum of my training I had to know how to stall a plane and recover as well as spin a plane and recover—both acrobatic maneuvers. True, these are the most basic of acro maneuvers, but acro they are! When you stall an airplane, it has nothing to do with an engine, (with few exceptions; gliders don't have engines anyway) but rather you stall the wings, stop them from producing lift, and you literally become like a rock falling from the sky with useless wings attached. A spin is the same thing as a stall, with the difference being the plane is induced into a spin at the entry of the stall. In both cases, the plane is in freefall.

So, once my doctor told me I wasn't allowed to do acro, I, of course, signed up within a few weeks for power plane acrobatic lessons at an airport near mine. I added four and a half hours of time in my logbook with those lessons and, by the end of that time, I could stall, spin (with far greater precision), loop, fly inverted, roll and barrel-roll an airplane. Of course, with that little time logged I wasn't an acro master, but I had mastered these maneuvers enough at the basic level, which was all I wanted. It really does something positive to your psyche to know you know how to toss an airplane around the sky.

Of course, I never told my doctor about this. Hey, I'm not suicidal!

My "past due date" had come and gone by several years. My suspicions that my heart had been improving were about to be proved correct, along with my strategies of bullying my heart and doing the opposite of what my doctor told me. Don't get me wrong, it's not as if I thought my doctor didn't know what he was doing. I'm still here, aren't I? He must've done things right, don't you think? Well, I certainly do. But I would have employed these strategies no matter who my doctor was. It came down to this: I was just listening to my heart. It always told me what to do or not do, and I always listened. Call it grace, Divine Inspiration, or just that my heart and I had this deep connection. No matter what you want to call it, I always listened to my heart. And my heart never lied.

Business was good and strong. I was involved in one of those great relationships I would later screw up. I was a pilot and still wasn't dead. Life was as good for me as it had ever been.

Shortly before my thirty-fourth birthday I had a doctor's visit. As always, they drew blood, gave me an EKG, my doctor conducting a thorough exam. This time he seemed quieter as he examined me and became more so when he was looking at the EKG read-out strip. Finally, he looked up from the strip and said, and these were his exact words, "I don't know how you did it, but your EKG is indistinguishable from a normal person's. You did it. You beat it. Go out and live."

A great big grin, filled with satisfaction, spread across his face. I jumped off the exam table and we shook hands vigorously.

I had been wanting to buy my own plane, but this news made the decision for me. I found a plane in Pennsylvania, not too far from Somerset, took one look, and fell in love. Went back another weekend with Al in tow, which is funny since Al was our tow pilot. Al inspected the plane and said it passed muster. So, on my thirty-fourth birthday, the seventeenth anniversary of my almost dying on my seventeenth birthday, I bought my own airplane to celebrate that, once again, I had beaten death, and at the same time I'd made my impossible dream come true.

58

The video production business started to change as the equipment continued to improve and reach the point that it was no longer necessary to know how to light or have the skill set previously necessary to work in a professional TV studio. The new video cameras and other equipment were making it so that even people without training could make passable video. Suddenly, "good enough" *really* became good enough, and sometimes not even good enough was deemed good enough. It seemed that as the equipment became better, the production standards became lower. On top of that, PowerPoint presentations were beginning to replace corporate videos, my bread and butter. And by now, corporate video had been discovered by the colleges, and they were pouring newly graduated students into the work and intern pool at a frantic rate. Unfortunately for those already in the biz, and the newbie's, these newcomers were too green, too eager, and too dim to realize that by cutting the rates of those of us already in the video business they were, in effect, also cutting their own throats. They eventually learned this, but it was too late for them when they realized what they had done, and the business as I'd known it was gone forever.

My friend, Larry, who had started with me in corporate video, had decided to move into entertainment some years back where he had to start at the bottom again. I, on the other hand, couldn't imagine that corporate video, as I'd known it, would ever change as radically as it did, so I wrongfully stayed the course. I've been out of that business for about 20 years now and Larry just won his fifteenth Emmy. But, as it would turn out, it all worked out for me in the end.

It was around this time that I met Rose through an ad I'd placed in the Penny Saver, a weekly publication for local businesses and individuals to advertise in. This was before the time of computer dating. I thought that a personal ad, placed in something as local as the Penny Saver, would be a good idea. It worked; Rose lived exactly one mile from my apartment. Neither of us had ever been married and to some minds we were late to the altar. But we didn't think so. I was thirty-seven and Rose was thirty-five, and that seemed fine to us.

We were married in seven months. She moved into my apartment, which was a big mistake. It was too small, and it never felt like "ours" as much as it felt like "mine," and it never really felt like "hers." We moved into the top floor of a two-family home, had wonderful landlords, and started building our life together.

With my brother Michael's help, we bought a puppy pug that we named Louie. Louie was Rose's starter dog, as it were, whereas I'd had dogs all my life. Up till then, Rose was terrified of dogs. I wish I'd made a video of the first time Rose met my sister's Great Dane. He wanted to say "Hi." He stood up, put his paws on Rose's shoulders so they could be face-to-face for their first meeting. Rose was so frightened she looked as if she had turned to stone. I think the Dane was disappointed that Rose turned out to be so uninteresting. Michael had a pug named Scoop, and it was Scoop who softened Rose's attitude enough for us to get a dog. Me? I wanted another German shepherd. I'd already had two, but Rose was going to have none of that. As it turned out, Louie was a blast, and we both fell in love with him, but he was a stubborn little thing. It took us ten months to get him to stop peeing around the house, at least for the most part.

I knew I had to do something about my business and started to cast around to see what else was out there. One night I received a phone call that led to a meeting at a hotel, and that got us interested in network marketing, also known as multi-level marketing (MLM). I had to start all over again, and it took me two years to get it off the ground, but once it was, it went great and started to build on itself. I had to work harder than I did in TV, but the payoff was better, and it had residual income to boot, something that we would be very grateful for in the near future.

We bought a house in Huntington, Long Island, in the hills and a short walk to either Huntington Bay on one side, or the Long Island Sound on the other. It had about half an acre, with gigantic 120 ft. pines in the backyard. Louie loved it. We loved it. Rose worked as a nurse, but that's not a fair description. Rose is an oncology nurse, and at that time, she was in charge of all cancer nursing for the largest hospital system in the state of New York. I was, and am, very proud of her, but she worked very hard, and I never liked that. Between us we were doing very well. As an offshoot of network marketing, I had also started a career as a public speaker, and that was doing well too. We had a nice house, two nice cars, and a pug who was still peeing all over the house. Who could ask for more? Life was grand. At least for a while.

I always maintained a good weight. When I got married, I

weighed about 136 pounds and kept that weight for the better part of ten years. But something was beginning to change with me and distant alarms, long silent, started to go off in my head. Almost any activity had me out of breath, and that was very unusual for me. I started to gain weight that I couldn't get rid of, also something that was very unusual for me. I went to my doctor. He immediately saw the weight gain, as my gut was hanging over my belt. I explained my symptoms and he ordered a blood test and an EKG. Nothing showed up on either, but to be sure he wanted me to wear a 24-hour halter, a portable EKG that they hooked me up to and that I wore for a complete day. I also had to take notes in a notebook that was provided listing all —and I mean *all*—activity that took place during that day, including the nature and time of the activity. Was I eating? Write it down. Was I watching TV? Write it down. Was I going to the bathroom? Write it down. Number one or two? Write it down. It was embarrassing. But, then again, what in medicine isn't? The way I look at it, not much.

When I returned to the doctor's, the test came back negative. Everything came back negative. My heart was ruled out as the cause of the shortness of breath and the weight gain I couldn't get rid of. Maybe I was just out of shape?

As those symptoms continued to progress, I was not paying as much attention to my business as I normally would have. One night, Joe Gentle and I were talking about the direction my business was heading, and I blurted I was worried about my heart. Joe was my upline, the person above me in the business, and by then a dear friend. Joe is one of the most honest people I have ever met, and based on what my doctor had told me, he thought I was being too dramatic or at least overly concerned. But that blurt had told me something; no, it was my heart telling me something, and my concern grew exponentially.

And something else started to happen, too. Our dog Louie became my shadow. He followed me everywhere, and honestly, he started to look worried. Something else in his behavior changed as well. Louie slept in bed with us, and he was allowed on the couch we used when we watched TV. He always liked to sleep in a crook of either of us; snuggled behind a bent knee, or against a bent thigh. But now he was sleeping almost exclusively against my chest, head against my heart, whether I was sitting or sleeping, and as the days went on he looked more and more worried.

Louie knew.

59

It is spring, in the year of 2000. I continued to get fatter and more out of breath. Diets that used to work like magic no longer had any effect. One day, I wanted to clear a brick path in the backyard, put there by the previous owner. There was no cement. He had just laid bricks on the bare ground and, over time, they had become more of a hazard than a walkway. I was 176 pounds. I was fat. I'd never been fat my entire life; actually, quite the opposite. I hardly recognized myself. Just bending down was difficult, let alone pulling the bricks from where they had settled into the stubborn earth and then tossing them into a wheelbarrow. In minutes I was gasping for breath. I hardly was able to stand and had to put one hand on the wheelbarrow for balance and the other was open-handed on my chest. I was doing my best impersonation of a guppy out of its fish bowl, flopping desperately for breath on the ground. Could I really be *this* out of shape? Every time I gasped for breath, it felt as if the air I was gulping contained no oxygen. Reason told me to stop what I was doing and just recover. I stumbled into the house and fell onto the couch. It took longer to recover than I would have expected. As soon as I hit the couch, I was joined by Louie, who looked at me with enormous concern, and then climbed onto my lap, sat, and put his head against my chest.

I told Rose a half version of the event, more as a way of explaining why most of the walkway was still there, as well as trying to stay in my current state of denial. *I'm just out of shape*, I kept telling myself. *I have to start an exercise program right away*. I was doing my best to ignore those distant alarms ringing in my head. After all, I'd been tested, and all the tests showed my heart was all right. And besides, I had a normal heart, right? That's what I'd been told. It couldn't be my heart. I was done with all of that, wasn't I? Wasn't I?

Then, on May 31, Larry came over so we could go on what we called a cigar walk. Cigars were very popular at that time, but I was no newbie. It wasn't a fad for me or for Larry. I'd been smoking high-quality cigars since I was sixteen. Larry and I both loved cigars, and we each maintained a first-rate stash of our own. We liked to go on walks in my neighborhood, which is hilly, without sidewalks, heavily wooded, and a short distance to a beach on Long Island Sound.

So, we set out on our walk, puffing away, but this time instead of heading to the beach we went in the opposite direction, up a fairly steep hill. We seldom took this route, but we just wanted a change. We weren't even halfway up the hill when I started to gasp for air. I was gasping as someone would if they had been underwater until the very last moment before they'd black out, but finally reached the surface at the last instant. My gasps had that same hollow sound as when I tried to pull up the brick walkway, and again they seemed to lack any oxygen. We were no more than a quarter mile from my house, but some of the way had a slight upward incline and my house was halfway up a very steep hill.

To put it bluntly, I scared the shit out of Larry. He wanted to get help, but I wouldn't allow it. Instead, I labored home, half walking, half being carried by Larry, heaving the entire way. Larry was bug-eyed with fright. It took a long time to finally get me home, and Larry wouldn't leave until I recovered, which also took a long time.

When Larry left, after he was sure I was all right, I called Rose and we both agreed I had to call my doctor. When I told him of the recent events, he immediately scheduled a stress test for the next day at Huntington Hospital, about a mile from my home.

On June 1st, at 8:00 a.m., I reported for my test. In a thallium stress test they insert an IV, inject thallium (a radioactive substance), have you wait for about half an hour or so, then have you scanned by a machine designed to pick up the radioactive signature of the thallium. This way they get a baseline of what your blood flow is as it travels through the heart. This test can also determine the ejection fraction of the heart, a measurement of how strongly the heart is pumping.

Once they have their baseline, they wire you up to an EKG and put you on a treadmill. Then they have you walk until your heartbeat reaches a certain value and rescan you again to note whatever changes occur when your heart is under stress. Well, that was the plan, anyway.

I tolerated the resting portion of the test with no difficulties, but now it was time for me to get on the treadmill. They wired me up (this test always makes me feel like a hamster in a lab experiment) and started the treadmill at a slow walking speed. I kept joking and acting as if I really didn't need to be there in the first place. But, inside I was nervous.

It didn't take long at all. In about 30 seconds, I started to collapse. The doctor and nurses rushed to catch me and slowly lowered me to the floor at the foot of the treadmill. Next thing I knew, I had an oxygen mask pressed to my face.

While I was being given oxygen, Rose was in another room being told her husband was in end-stage heart failure. I was forty-six years old.

60

I went home that day after I recovered. I remember it being a beautiful day. Sometime in mid-afternoon, my home office phone rang. It was my doctor calling to give me the findings from that morning. He was somber. The news wasn't good. First, he told me I was in complete heart block. Again, the signal from my brain to my heart was being blocked, incapacitating the heart's ability to pump blood to the rest of the body.

Also, I had congestive heart failure—*failure* being the key word here. There is no cure, the heart is failing, and on its way to coming to a complete stop. Forever. So, what's the answer? The only cure for heart failure, he explained, is a heart transplant. *A transplant!* I felt my world coming apart around me as the implications of that word started to sink in. My vision became very narrow and all else seemed to blur. I knew at that moment that nothing would be the same ever again. And it never was.

Also, he told me, I was to be admitted to North Shore University Hospital in the morning.

Some other things were said before we hung up shortly afterwards, but I couldn't tell you what they were. I was numb and felt like I was melting right into the floor. Nothing seemed real anymore. I'd been standing during the phone call, but I just fell into my chair, crossed my arms on my desk, dropped my head in my arms and said to myself, *Oh no, it's starting again. It's starting again!* I began to weep, from the depths of my soul, weep. I was not crying because I'd just been given a possible death sentence. Compared to why I was crying, death didn't mean that much to me. I was crying because I knew I was in for a long haul of nurses and doctors and hospital stays, where they would cut, poke, and stick me, put me in machines, strip me of my dignity, and ultimately cause me a great deal of pain. Oh, I'm sorry; doctors, hospitals and nurses never put a patient in pain, they only make them "uncomfortable."

I cried for no more than five minutes, and when I was done, I was done. I gathered myself, got up, went to Rose and told her the news. She looked devastated, and other than that I can't remember anything about the rest of that day or night. That would be the only time I cried about my current condition. From that day on, I never shed so much as a single tear over my predicament. Not one. I was already getting ready for this, my latest battle, and you can't be an effective soldier if you are looking at the world through your own tears. It keeps you from seeing clearly and can cause you to use the wrong strategy. Crying for yourself can take the fight out of you and make you start to feel sorry for yourself, a prescription for death, in my way of thinking. Of course, I wasn't in full warrior mode yet, not by a long shot, but I had started to armor-up. The next day, I said goodbye to Louie, who looked as if he'd heard and understood every word my doctor told me over the phone the previous day. It broke my heart. I think he thought he'd never see me again.

Rose drove me to the hospital where I was admitted for shortness of breath, complete heart block and congestive heart failure. It had begun.

61

On June 2nd, I was admitted to North Shore, in the same building where Rose ran the chemo unit. I didn't feel well because they had given me Nitro paste, a form of nitroglycerin, and almost immediately it produced an intense headache. That is a common effect of this drug, as is the nausea and vomiting that followed it. I was given Tylenol, but because it didn't help too much, they upped the ante and gave me Percocet, which helped more, but I still had a low-grade headache all the same.

That night, at about 8:00 p.m., I was taken to the Cardiac Catheterization Lab. I have to admit, I was afraid of this procedure, seeing how much pain and nightmares went with the one I had just prior to my seventeenth birthday. To my great relief, this was three decades later and medical science had advanced quite a bit since then. The doctor who was to perform the test was the head of the lab. He was a good-looking man with salt and pepper hair (mostly salt) and a neatly trimmed beard to match. He was

friendly and gentle and spoke to me through most of the procedure, I think, to help calm me down, which it did. His touch
was gentle, and the procedure was almost painless compared to
my last cath.

Once he had the catheter in place and was able to get a good
look inside my arteries and heart he said, "Your arteries are
crystal clear. I thought we'd have to put a stent in you. When you
get out of here you can celebrate at a steakhouse!" But that wasn't
everything he found; *that* info he shared with Rose.

That time when I was speaking with my upline, Joe, when I
had told him I was worried about my heart, was not the first
time I gave voice to the distant alarms my heart was sounding.
The first time I said anything to Rose was two years previously. I
remember we were talking and I had said to her, "I think I'm
going to need a new heart soon." Rose turned on me and said,
"Where do you get these ideas?" She was almost mad at me for
saying it.

But now Rose was in the doctor's office and he told her my
heart was enlarged, quite enlarged, and that I had idiopathic
cardiomyopathy, a wasting disease of the heart caused by an
unknown agent. Your husband, he told her, is going to need a
heart/lung transplant. Rose instantly burst into tears, and told
the doctor, "Oh my God, he tried to tell me, and I didn't believe
him!" There it was. I needed both a heart and a pair of lungs. In
no way was any of this good news, and, in no way did that mean
it couldn't get worse.

Very early the next day I was taken from my room to another
procedure room to have an Electro Physiology Study, or EPS.
This test was to determine the electrical functionality of my heart.
It was typical of any procedure room: all white, nurses and techs
scurrying around getting ready for the next procedure, which in

this case was mine. I really don't remember that test, but a few hours after it was over, and I was back in my room, a young, handsome doctor who brought with him an air of kindness mixed with humor entered. He wanted to talk about the results of the EPS. I motioned for him to sit on my bed, and he did. I liked him instantly. His name was Dr. Park. He was a Korean American doctor who was as Korean as I am Italian, which pretty much means in heritage only. There was just something about him that made me glad he was in my room. Although, as it had been with every doctor I'd dealt with in the last few days, I had serious doubts if he was there just to chat casually.

As I had expected, based on the fact that he had sat on the bed and wanted to talk to me, I knew the results from the EPS were not going to be good. I was right. They weren't good at all. As a matter of fact, they were quite grim. The bottom line came down to this: I needed a pacemaker and I needed it now. I think that Dr. Park had been able to size me up the same way I had him. He spoke calmly, and for the most part, wore a warm smile when it was appropriate.

When he was done telling me about the need for a pacemaker, I told him I didn't want one. But he said I needed one, to which I replied, and this next bit of our conversation is exact quotes: "Dr. Park, I resisted a pacemaker for all the years that my doctor wanted me to have one, and I resist one now." He just sat on the bed, nodded his head up and down a little and thought for a bit. Then he turned to me and said, "Your EKG is incompatible with life." It took me a moment or two to digest and interpret what he had just said. When its full meaning finally dawned behind my stubbornness, I said, "Oh! So, when can we do this?" In just a few minutes with me Dr. Park had figured out exactly how to tell me something in a way I wouldn't fight and could understand completely. I will never forget that man and I will always be grateful to him.

Well, as it turned out, they already had me scheduled for a pacemaker insertion at 8:00 the next morning. That's when the cutting would begin.

62

As planned, they came for me the next morning and took me to the room where the insertion/ installation would take place. Again, one could hear the *clink* and *tinkle* of surgical instruments being laid out. Sometimes, I thought they almost sounded like wind chimes. Against one wall was a massive machine, big enough to put me into, which, of course, they did. It kind of looked like a giant white barrel laid on its side with the side and top cut open. To the left was the end of the barrel, with a hole in it at the bottom for my head to go through. Once inside this thing it felt like I was in a heart-lung machine, because all I could see was this great big white metal wall in front of my face. I could see into the room, off at an angle, but I couldn't see the rest of me or what they were doing to me. On the other hand, they could see me from the neck down, but they were unable to see my face.

You have to understand just how terrified I was at that point. I thought I had beaten this thing. I thought all the cutting and pain were things of the past. Yet, there I was with a "disembodied head" staring at this huge white metal wall, not even able to watch what they were doing. I would have no indication of what they were about to do, and thus no way to at least prepare myself a little for what was coming next. The fact that it was starting all over again was my worst nightmare, and this was only the beginning of what I knew was going to be a long and painful road.

They had given me a mild sedative, and the placement of the pacemaker was going to be done using local anesthetics. They were going to make a "pocket" out of the muscle of my upper chest wall to give the pacemaker a place to reside. They were also going to add a support section to the artery and then thread two thin cables through that support and artery into my heart. The cables would then be located permanently in my heart using the self-tapping screws at the end of each cable that would screw into the heart muscle itself.

The sedative did nothing for the tremendous anxiety I was experiencing. I can't remember a single time in my life when I was so anxious; well, *damned scared*. I was stiff as a board with fright. I was so stiff, you could have used my body as a bridge between two points. When I realized just how rigid I was, a tiny part of my rationality appeared. *Okay*, I said to myself, *you're stiff as a board. All of your muscles are tremendously tensed and that can't be good for the surgery. It can only hurt you. Okay, okay, I have to relax. But how?* Then I said to myself, *Why not start by saying the Lord's Prayer?*

So, I did, silently to myself, but I don't think I ever said it with as much emotion and conviction as I did then. That seemed to help. Now what? I know a lot of people would, at that point, have asked for something: Please make the operation go well; please don't let it hurt; and so on. But I couldn't do that. I've always had this feeling—and I know a lot of people don't share this sentiment, and that's fine—but I just don't believe I can ask

God for things. He's not my butler. It's quite the other way around, I think. We are supposed to be instruments of *His* will; what business do I have in asking *Him* for something? Well, that's what I believe, anyway. We're all unique and this is just the way *I* deal with God. You believe what you believe; you'll get no argument from me.

So, I started thinking. I was supposed to be dead when I was five, then again at six. I wasn't supposed to make it past ten, but I did. Then I almost died on my seventeenth birthday, and the next few days after, but Divine Intervention had taken care of me instead. Then I wasn't supposed get out of my twenties, and yet at the age of thirty-three I was told I'd beaten the whole thing. I'm a pilot, owned my own television production company, and a marketing business. I had a beautiful home complete with a beautiful wife and a pug that peed all over. And there I was after all of that at age forty-six, an age no gambler would have ever bet that I'd attain. Best of all, I'd lived more in my forty-six years than most who live into their eighties did! In all the ways that truly counted, I was a wealthy man.

And so, I started to get grateful. Down-to-the-bottom-of-my-soul grateful. As I re-counted all that I just stated and gave my deepest thanks for each and every one of them, something wondrous happened. I suddenly felt a presence, not of one individual, but of many. Then I heard it, a chorus of voices sang "Ahhhhhhhhh." It was unbelievably beautiful. I knew instantly what it was that I had just heard. It was the chorale, the chorus of angels. And then I became filled with a warmth, which is as close as I'll ever get in describing it. This warmth not only filled me but surrounded me, held me, *assured me*. Next thing I knew, I was being flooded, downright *flooded* with the purest love I had ever known. It was *miraculous* in the most literal sense of the word, and all my fears completely vanished. My stark terror had been replaced with joy and bliss and this incredible, all-consuming feeling of love. I was loved, and I wasn't alone and was being told in no uncertain terms. Tears of joy were streaming down my face. It was incredibly beautiful. I'd go through everything I'd ever been through before—all the pain, the suffering and fear all over again—just to re-live that moment. It was one of the most powerful experiences I ever had in my entire life, second only to my NDE. I'd been given another gift. I was overflowing with gratitude, gratitude for every single thing that had ever happened to me in my life—good or bad. It was an epiphany, and it changed my life, especially how I would handle the wait for an organ and the transplant itself.

From that moment on, all the way through to the end of transplant, I had no fears of *anything*. I was in a place of peace and serenity. I cherished my latest gift and lived in the attitude of gratitude that had been infused into me by the members of that chorale. And who knows, maybe The Voice had something, or everything, to do with this as well.

And the surgery? I didn't feel a thing from the moment on that I'd heard those angelic voices.

63

I was still having intense pain in my abdomen. The same day as the implantation of the pacemaker, I also had a sonogram of my abdomen, a liver function test, and a kidney function test. When the results came back they were surprising, almost shocking. Here's the rundown: I was in complete heart block. I had congestive heart failure. I was in lung failure. I had sludge in my gall bladder, and my liver and kidneys where in partial failure. All of this was really the result of the congestive heart failure. The other organs were beginning to fail because the heart was failing. I guess it was some sort of organic chain reaction. Bottom line was that if I hadn't collapsed with Larry, or told my doctors about it, I would have been dead in but a few days or weeks. I wasn't out of the woods yet, but at least I gotten back on the path that would temporarily lead me out from under their canopy.

After this complete diagnosis was made, I was moved into the Cardiac Care Unit. Here they started me on Dobutamine, a drug meant to help my heart pump more effectively, and IV

Lasix, a diuretic to help get all the water weight off me. Sometimes known as water pills, diuretics are used to increase the production of urine.

When someone has congestive heart failure, the heart is losing its ability to pump efficiently. Because of this, the afflicted retains a lot of water because the heart isn't sending enough blood to the kidneys, fluid builds up in the belly, the bottom of the legs, and especially in the ankles and the pericardial sac, the bag-like membrane that surrounds the heart. This, of course, puts even more pressure on the heart, making it harder and harder to be able to beat. It is easy to see how this vicious cycle can lead to death. In the time of one week, I lost 30 pounds of water weight as a result of being on IV Lasix. One of the reasons my condition wasn't caught earlier was because I carried no water in my legs. It all went to my belly. It is not common at all for someone with heart failure as advanced as mine to not have swollen ankles. If they had been swollen, my condition would have made itself known much earlier.

The next day they changed my drugs around a bit, and I met with a cardiologist. This was my life for the next few days. Then on June 13th, I was transferred out of the CCU to a hospital room. My spirits were high but ever since that walk with Larry, my body wasn't the same. It was as if that walk had thrown a switch and now my body had been put into "sick mode." I was weak, couldn't walk too fast or far, and was always tired.

Finally, on June 15th, 2000, I was *discharged*. Well, that's hospital terminology. I prefer to say I was *released* from NSUH and free to go home. I'd survived the opening salvo of my new challenge. I'd won that battle, but the war was just getting started. I didn't care. That would all be dealt with soon enough, but for then all that mattered was I was going home. *Home!*

When we arrived, Rose parked in the driveway. Our house is

built into a hill and the front door is grade level. We have a high-ranch, so when you step into the house, you can take six steps up to the main level, of which, if you walked to the back of the main level, to the deck off the kitchen, it's a full story above ground level. If Rose had parked in back, I would have had to walk up twelve steps instead of six. The layout of the house would play a more and more important role in my life as the disease progressed.

Rose thought it would be a good idea if she went and got Louie and brought him out to me. In the time it took Rose to go down the walkway, open the door, gather Louie and bring him out to me, all I'd been able to do was to get halfway up the walkway. When Louie saw me, he exploded with excitement. He was in Rose's arms, about three feet from me and he tried to jump the distance. We both believe he thought I had died and that he'd never see me again.

Oh, God, it was good to have Louie in my arms again.

64

This was the start of another new life for me. I would be going to doctors at *least* once a week; exams, blood tests, this doctor, that doctor, this drug change, that drug change. If I gave a blow-by-blow account of all the visits it would be as interesting as the book of Genesis is in the Bible; that is to say, not too much. But during that time, I met with the cardiologist I'd met at North Shore. He told me I shouldn't be worried, that my condition wasn't too bad and could be kept under control with drugs. He also stated that he thought I had about ten years before I'd have to worry about a transplant. Well, *that* was certainly good news, wasn't it?

But my house was beginning to become a prison for me. Other than for doctor visits, I was pretty much staying home. I had turned my business over to my upline, Joe Gentle, and he ran it honestly and vigorously for me throughout the entire time up to transplant and after. It was one less thing to worry about, and something I will always be grateful for. I was pretty much spending the entire day in our family room, on the lower level, watching TV with Louie. I learned quickly that even with the best cable package there is nothing, *nothing*, worth watching on TV during the daytime hours.

But I wasn't just sitting there like a lump. I was actively thinking of ways to armor-up, of strategies to cope, and how to lessen the impact on Rose. I had the thought that neither of us should take that journey on our own, that it would be a good idea if we had professional help– guides, if you will—who could help us navigate that particular passage. So, I contacted an MSW, master's in social work, a therapist, to help us. I had insisted that Rose do the same thing. Rose is an absolute master in the skills of denial. I think she has a black belt in it, but I knew she needed some sort of guidance as well. As it turned out, the therapist I'd contacted was married to a therapist. Rose went to her and I started weekly sessions with him. It was a good move, and we both benefited as a result.

All that time, Rose, being the nurse that she was, had been casting for a second opinion. She wanted the best and recalled that she had a friend from North Shore who was working in the heart failure department of Columbia Presbyterian Hospital. Rose contacted her and was told she worked directly with a doctor who was considered, depending on who you spoke with, the number one or two heart-failure specialist in the world. Just what Rose was looking for. Through her friend we were able to get an appointment quickly.

I will never forget this, and I know neither will Rose. We went to visit her on June 18th, 2000. The transplant/heart failure unit was a converted section of what used to be a hospital patient floor, with converted patient rooms now exam rooms. The central nurses' station of the unit was now reception.

We went to the exam room the doctor was in and made our introductions. She sat at a tiny desk and was paging through a thick file; my file. It took her a couple of moments before she stopped reading, lifted her head, and looked at me. After another moment or two of looking me over, she said, "You were told you have about ten years, right?"

"Yes," I replied.

"You're lucky if you have one."

And that's how I met the woman who would save my life.

Her prognosis, as we would find out, was almost exact. I don't know why there was such a disparity between the two doctors, hers and the one from North Shore. Was he just trying to comfort me, or had he misread the situation? I'm afraid I'll never know, but I do know I hold no ill will towards him. In either case, I'm certain he was sincere and doing his best for me. You can't complain about that.

My new doctor told me I had to start to limit my fluid intake to 40 ounces a day and to eliminate as much salt from my diet as possible. Fluids, by the way, meant all fluids: fruit, soups, vegetables, anything with water content had to count in my daily 40 ounces. Previously, my cardiologist had told me that salt and water were my enemies. I really took it to heart. At my last North Shore hospitalization, I was given a booklet from the AHA, American Heart Association, that listed the salt content in foods. It was amazingly complete. Did you know that ice cream and candy bars contain salt? Did you know there is salt in the tap water you drink? I certainly didn't.

For me, the only way to track things like that was to make a list. First, I had been an on-and-off-again juicer, I already had a good idea of the water content of a lot of fruits and vegetables. But to be sure, so I could keep an accurate count, I juiced a single carrot and measured how much juice—water really—it yielded. I wrote it down and then did that for all the fruits and vegetables that I normally ate. Then I got a plastic pitcher, marked in ounces, measured 40 ounces, and drew a line around the pitcher to indicate that amount and make it easy for me to see.

I started my list: I wrote down every single thing I ate in a day, including the salt content of the food. Every morning, I would fill the pitcher exactly with forty ounces of fresh water. If I ate a piece of fruit, I would subtract that amount from my pitcher. At the end of each day I would write down how much my fluid intake was for that day.

If you are on water and/or salt restrictions, the above is an excellent way to keep yourself on track. Hey, your life might depend on it.

I'm pretty much a slob. My office looks like a bomb hit it. It drives Rose nuts. But that's the way I am, and I know precisely where everything is in the mess. "Ordered Chaos" I've been told it's called. But when I get my mind set to something I become very ordered in that particular thing, hence the lists. I'm also very disciplined. When I'm on a mission, I can't be swayed. Water and salt were my enemy? Then that's how I would treat them. I'm only allowed 40 ounces of fluids a day? Well then, I'll do better than that. I was averaging, in ounces, in the low 30's. Some days, I was in the mid-20's. I was dying of thirst, my mouth was always dry, but I didn't care. I was in *battle*.

I didn't know yet that I had made a serious mistake. Doctors, from experience, know that patients often lie to them. Diabetics tell doctors they have cut down on sugar but have multiple doughnuts, beer and pasta every day. Patients tell doctors they are exercising daily when they haven't gotten off the couch in a month. I didn't know that many patients don't tell the truth to their doctors. Me? I'm a hyper-compliant patient, and they didn't know that about me. I tell the truth and assumed everyone else did in matters as serious as life and death.

Soon, this miscommunication would become a very big deal.

65

On July 26th, I started three days of testing at Columbia for my eligibility to be on the transplant list. It was three days of physical tests and, the one I dreaded, mental tests. Those truly were the ones I was afraid I would fail, but I passed them, as well as the rest.

Why do they test for eligibility? For several reasons and all of them are valid. Physically, they have to know you don't have any other diseases, such as cancer, that would make giving you an organ—pardon my bluntness—a waste. America is generally a very generous country, always first to help other countries in a disaster and the home of countless charities. Even neighbor to neighbor, we are unbelievably charitable, except when it comes to organ donation. We have a news media that stubbornly continues to be misinformed about the issue and gives no indication that it will educate itself. We have an entertainment media that constantly tells stories that support the myths and misconceptions about donation, thus scaring the average person from signing-up as a donor. The result of all of this translates to a terrible shortage in available organs, and *19 –20* people die every day in America because an organ didn't get to them in time. It's shameful, really. A true national disgrace. I believe with all my heart that if America was disabused of all the myths and misconceptions that surround organ donation, there would be no shortage of organs. Wouldn't that be a blessed thing?

But the general population isn't so disabused. That's why organs are few and precious. Doctors *have* to be very careful as to who gets them. If there is another disease process in a patient's body that will kill either the organ or the patient, then they have to be deemed as ineligible. That organ *has* to go to someone who can get full use of it. Believe me, if I had been found ineligible, I would not have argued. How could I? It would have been an immensely selfish act, wouldn't it?

As far as the psychiatric exam, they had to be sure that if you were given an organ you would take care of it properly. I was told that Columbia had a patient a long time ago who, after receiving his heart, just disappeared. No follow-up, no figuring out the cocktail of drugs that would keep him alive. They can only assume he died a short while after, taking that precious heart, a heart that could have saved someone who would have made good use of it, with him. After that, they started the psychiatric protocol, which I agree with 100 percent. Again, these organs, all the transplantable organs, are rare and precious.

When you are given the Gift of Life, as it is often called, you are being given not just a new chance of life, but an immense responsibility as well. It is up to the individual given the gift to maintain and nurture it. It is the least you can do for the donor who gave it to you, as well as for his/her family. In a sense, they gave it, too, and that piece of their loved one that you are walking around with is not only a part of you, but a part of that family as well. It is most humbling.

The distance from the parking lot to the part of Columbia that did transplants was not a full city block. But it was uphill; not steep, but uphill. At this stage I was able to "tolerate activity," as they would say medically, but not much of it. When I was going for those three days of tests, I had to stop multiple times each day to catch my breath and regain the strength to continue. It was not much of a hill, but to me it was just slightly shy of Mt. Everest.

I was also experiencing terrible leg cramps, usually in the morning or at night. They were unbelievably painful, and when I got cramps in my ankles, it felt as if someone was trying to separate my foot from my ankle with a butter knife.

On August 4th my doctor presented and made my case at the transplant board, and I was officially placed on the list. I was listed as a "2," but my doctor didn't think that was the right category for me. As the listings were then, you could get listed as a 1A, which meant you were very sick, in desperate need of a heart, and currently hospitalized. A 1B meant you are very sick but could be home. Being a 2 meant you're sick and home, but the chances of being given an organ at that stage are very unusual. During my three days of testing I did a type of stress test where the person administrating the test pushed me almost to the point of collapse. My doctor thought that skewed the overall results in the wrong direction.

Either way, it was official; I was going to get a heart transplant if I could get one in time. Now, all I had to do was wait and stay alive long enough to get one.

66

This was the beginning of the official wait for the organ. If the time I collapsed with Larry on our "cigar walk" is included with the time of the wait, the entire process took a year. During that time, I was hospitalized numerous times, both at Columbia and North Shore. I had to go to the emergency room multiple times, as well. I think it would be beyond boring to recount all those instances, but several events during the wait stand out and are pertinent to the story.

I was doing everything I could to prepare myself mentally for the outcome, whether it was a successful transplant, or I was finally going to get to meet The Voice. I was still deeply under the influence from that moment when I heard the chorus, and, if anything, the influence of that experience grew deeper every minute. I was in an incredibly "Zen" place, as I like to describe it. I had no fear, none whatsoever, on whatever outcome – life or death – was to be. Was I still afraid of pain? Yeah, but not as much. And after a while, barely at all. I had reached this place of what I called, "walking the 50/50 line." Fifty percent of me was prepared for the chance of survival and all I'd have to do to adjust to being a transplant. The other fifty percent of me was ready to die. It was absolutely 50/50—not 49/51 or 51/49. I was in a state of peace and serenity that before this I'd never even known was possible.

That attitude had been cemented into me shortly after I'd heard the chorus. I was at my brother-law Joe's house, sitting with him outside, and he wanted to know how I was doing. I didn't tell him about hearing those heavenly voices, but instead I shared with him what I had learned from the experience. I was supposed to be dead at five, I told him, then at six. I was never supposed to get past ten and then I had almost died on my seventeenth birthday. I wasn't supposed get out of my twenties and yet I had, and in the process had become a television production person with his own business and—more recently—a new business that was also going well. I had fulfilled my impossible dream of becoming a pilot and had owned my own airplane. I had a beautiful wife and home, complete with a pug that peed all over it. How could I be upset about any of that? I was supposed to die so many times and yet there I was, forty-six years old—still here. It was all gravy, I told him. It was all gravy. If now was the time when I was supposed to go, the only emotion I could feel about it was gratitude.

And therein lies the secret. I think it's the secret to life, but it's difficult to follow. You have to be grateful for everything. I mean *everything*. The Bible tells us "to be grateful in all things," *all* being the operative word. What good is it to only be grateful when things are going your way? There is no accomplishment in that. But to be grateful when things are against you, well now, *that's* really something. My mother died in my arms a year after my transplant—and I was grateful. Why do you have to be grateful when things happen that are bad for you? Because we are each just one thread in an infinite tapestry. We can't see anything more than the threads that immediately surround us. We have no idea, not the smallest scintilla of a clue, of what that tapestry is or what it represents. What I believe, and you don't have to agree with me, is that every one of us is here on our own personal journey. We each follow a unique path; a path that is ours alone. We die when we are supposed to die—even if we're murdered—because we have walked our particular path and have come to the end of our journey. We have accomplished what we were supposed to. So, when an obstacle is thrown in my face, I believe I have to be grateful for it because it is a part of the path I alone must walk. I believe in this deeply, and lately, I have to admit, it's sometimes difficult to summon the strength to be grateful at all times. But during the time of the wait, and for some time after, it was my natural way. I still feel 50/50 about death, but I struggle lately to return to that "Zen" place that got me through the pain, and sometimes agony and boredom, that those eight months were.

Being trapped all day in front of a television that offered nothing substantial to watch gave me an immense amount of time to think. Not only did I think about all that I was grateful for, I often thought of my donor, if I was to have one, which always unsettled me. At that point I was not as educated on transplantation as I am now, but I knew that for a heart to be viable, the donor's death is often caused by a sudden trauma: gunshot, fall of some kind, a beating or a car accident, just to name a few. It occurred very early during my wait how unfair this was. I was sick, literally deathly sick. I knew my condition without a transplant was terminal. I had all the time in the world, when compared to my donor, if I wasn't going to get one, to make peace with myself, God, Rose, and my friends. My donor, on the other hand, would have no idea that he/she, was about to die. They, and all donors, would have no idea they had just awakened and gotten out of bed for the last time. They would have no idea it was the last time they were going to have breakfast, lunch, or dinner; put on socks; apply lipstick; kiss or hug their loved ones. They had no idea their plans for the weekend, upcoming vacation, or new job interview, was never going to happen. No, the donor would be all right one moment and then in the next their life would be taken away. It just didn't seem fair. They'd have no chance to come to terms with things or prepare in any way as I did. To the donor, it was always a sudden shock. When I thought this way, I would wish I could time travel and get in the way of whatever was about to hit them and take the hit myself. But things don't work that way. I sometimes even thought it might be better if I just died. But then I'd think whatever was supposed to happen to them would still happen regardless if I was dead or alive, and I would mentally slump with helpless frustration.

So, I vowed to myself that if I were to get an organ I would take the best care of it as I could. I owed the donor and his family at least that much, I thought. Then I would think if I got the heart, that would mean someone else on the list who was slightly less sick than myself wouldn't get it. And if that was the case, there was no guarantee they'd get the chance at another before they became too sick to receive it or simply died while waiting. That made me realize that if I did get a heart I would be responsible to both the donor and the patient who didn't get it.

Little did I know that thoughts like those were the seeds for the survivor's guilt that would follow.

67

I take active survival strategies very seriously. Combined with how much time I had on my hands, I was considering all aspects of my current situation and finding ways to deal with them.

I'd heard that patients can hear while they are under anesthesia, they just don't remember it. Oddly enough, Columbia had done experiments about that theory and proved it true. So, I got the idea of making a CD of music for me to listen to in the operating room, if I was to be lucky enough to receive a heart. I asked my friend Mark to make me a "heart CD." I made a list of songs, put them in the order I wanted, and Mark made me the CD.

I cannot tell you how crucial this CD became during the period of the wait. At one of my visits to Columbia a male physical therapist had told me to think of my energy as money in a wallet and that every day would start with that wallet full. Everything I did, he said, was taking money out of that wallet and I'd want to do my best not to go "broke" on any particular day. He was exactly right. I'd reached the point where I could only go up and down the stairs once a day. I had to be sure where I wanted to spend what part of what day where. Our bedroom and my office are on the first floor. If I wasn't downstairs watching TV, I was in my office playing computer games or surfing the Net. So, when in my office, I played that CD over and over. I never played it if I was feeling blue, as I only wanted to associate it with positive feelings. Each song would take me to a different place and it became a great way for me to escape.

I had another reason for the CD. I knew that when I went in for the operation, I wasn't going to know a single person in the room. And they wouldn't know me from a hole in the wall. I didn't like that; I used the CD as a way for them to get to know me. If you listen to all the songs, and paid attention, I was telling whoever was listening who I was. There were songs that were meant for the doctors, songs that were meant for Rose, and songs that were meant for me. I even made it clear to the doctors that if I died, it would be all right. For some reason, it was important for the doctors to know who I was, and that I was more than just another transplant operation. I wanted them to know *I* was there too, not just my body.

There I'd sit, night after night in front of my computer, playing my heart CD while happily playing games, girding myself for what could possibly come. That wasn't the only time I played the CD, either. As a heart failure patient, I had to go to Columbia once every two weeks. Rose and I called it "going to the spa." As you already know, I am an avid car nut and driving a car, especially one with a stick, was and is one of my favorite things to do. The car I had then, as with my current cars, had a stick shift. So, going to the spa gave me the chance to get out of the house, drive a stick, and listen to my CD, which we did every single time we went. Rose and I always acted as if we were going someplace fun on those visits and would sing along with the songs as we drove. The CD was a powerful way for me to keep my spirits up, and since I never played it when I was down, just hearing it always made me feel good.

This is the list of the songs on that CD and why I picked them. None of them have ever felt or sounded the same since. I have provided a key to make it easier.

Key:

D = to the doctors

S = to me

R = to Rose

DN = to my donor and his family

1. *Help* - The Beatles D

Obviously, I needed help and wanted the doctors to know I was coming to them for it. Listen to the words, they take on a whole new meaning.

2. *Spirit in the Sky* - Norman Greenbaum D, S, R

I was all right, no matter what the outcome.

3. *If I Only Had a Heart* – Tin Man from the Wizard of Oz D

A joke to the doctors.

4. *I left My Heart in San Francisco* - Tony Bennett S

Private joke between my best friend, Concetta, and me. We called it, "I Left My Heart on the Transplant Table."

• • •

5. *My Heart Will Go On* - Celine Dion R, DN

I know, I know. This one used to make my ears bleed too, but while I was waiting, I heard it and suddenly it was appropriate for Rose, my donor and his family.

6. *PIANO CONCERTO NO. 5, "EMPEROR"* - Beethoven S, D

My favorite piece of music on this earth. The musical embodiment of triumph over adversity.

7. *I've Got You Under My Skin* - Dianna Krall D

"I've got you, deep in the heart of me" And what a voice!

8. *Ain't That a Kick in the Head?* - Dean Martin D, R, S

So upbeat it's contagious. "If I felt any better I'd be sick." One of my favorite big band arrangements.

9. *Oh Bla Dee* - Beatles S, R, D

Obvious. Fun, too.

10. *The Shoop-Shoop Song* - Cher S, R

One for Rose and me.

11. *High Hopes* - Frank Sinatra S, R, D

It's just the way I felt.

12. *Start All Over Again* - Dianna Krall S, R, DN

Same thing. It's how I've always thought about life.

13. *When I'm 64* - Beatles S, R, D

Just knew I would make it. We also believed, at the time, one couldn't get a transplant after age 64.

14. *Heart And Soul* - Ella Fitzgerald S, R, D

Hey, it's Ella.

15. *Young At Heart* - Jimmy Durantee S, R, D, DN

The theme song of my life. What can I say? I'm a Toys R Us kid. Also, Jimmy was a friend of my father's.

16. *You've Gotta Have Heart* - Damn Yankees S, L

A thank you to my donor and his family to let him know without him and their generosity I wouldn't have anything. I'm eternally grateful.

But things weren't rosy for Rose. One of the things I was constantly aware of was that the whole situation had to be harder on her than it was for me. Of course, Rose did have her super-powers to protect her, her great abilities of denial, but they only went so far. The reality was that Rose was watching her husband in the process of dying, and every day there was a little less of me there. That was a great concern for me, and sometimes I would speak to her as we were lying in bed. I'd tell her what kind of funeral I wanted so she wouldn't have to guess, if that was what was to be. I said I wanted to be an organ/tissue donor. I told her, over and over again, that if I died, I wanted her to know I was all right, that I've had so much gravy in my life and that I wanted her to be as grateful as was I. I told her I wanted her to move on if I died, and that I'd only be happy if she was happy too. I made her promise me on that one, but Rose being the Italian she is, I wouldn't be surprised if, after my death, she wore a black dress for the rest of her life! But I was doing everything I could to make sure Rose would be okay if anything happened to me. I'd said I never cried about this situation after that one time when my doctor told me the results of the stress test. It's true; I never cried about my own situation. But I did cry when I thought of Rose. The idea of how much that would hurt her had me weeping silently next to her in bed, at least once a week.

Toward the end, Rose's super-powers were finally defeated. During the last few months of the wait, I had become so sick that I could hardly move. Up to that point I was doing three things every day. I was cooking dinner, which almost daily caused me to go shopping. Okay, it took me a long time to shop, but I could get out of the house and while I walked the supermarket aisles I could at least lean on the shopping cart. Cooking itself wasn't bad because all I had to do was stand there and prepare the meals. The second thing I did every day was to make the bed. It took three times longer than it took normally, but it gave me something to do, and I thought at least it was something to lift some of the burden from Rose. The third thing I did was bring the empty garbage pails in after they were put out for trash pick-up, until the day came when I couldn't.

Again, our house is built into a hill, with street level being higher than the house level. To get the pails I'd have to walk up a three-foot grade. The day finally came when that walk became impossible for me. Rose told me after the transplant that when she came home from work and saw that the pails hadn't been taken in, it was like a smack in the head. She realized why they were still there, and she turned her car around and drove for 45 minutes crying. She seldom cried in front of me about my condition, but she had to cry so much, and for so long, she didn't want me to see it or know it.

Rose's super-power had finally been defeated, and oddly, those pails turned out to be her kryptonite.

68

When I was first diagnosed I was told I'd need both a heart and lungs. But I'd been hyper-compliant with my water and salt intake, and one day I was given the news that they no longer thought I needed new lungs. As a result of my taking as little water as I did, however, I'd become dangerously dehydrated; so dehydrated that about 50 percent of my alveoli—the little cauliflower-looking things in your lungs that make the passage of oxygen to the blood possible —had burst. So, I saved my lungs but permanently lost 51 percent of my lung function in the process. I can't quite remember if this was the same time that I threw a blood clot in my lungs, but I'm pretty sure it was. This resulted in two things: another hospitalization and getting taken off the transplant list because I was no longer healthy enough to receive a heart. I was kept off the list for about six weeks until the issue was resolved.

They did a procedure called an "A-line," where they go into an artery through the wrist to measure the gas levels in the blood. Problem was, it wouldn't stop bleeding once they were done. I bled for hours, with them putting one bandage on only to replace it with the next one. Each bandage, which was basically a large gauze roll, compressed and held in place with white tape, lasted only minutes. This was bad, and they were quite upset. It wasn't until late in the night that it finally stopped bleeding. The nurse, who was with me at that time changing one bandage after another, was frantic. This caused a real scare for her. I guess it would have scared me, too, if I'd been in her position. But I wasn't too concerned. Deep in my Zen zone, I figure.

As you can imagine, the stress levels at home were high, and both Rose and I started to express that stress in an unusual way. At night, in bed, we became the farting twins. I mean full brass section, loud as a trombone farts. It was comical, even to us. We quickly got into the habit of saying, "Sorry," after the latest blast, and that became a private joke that often cracked us up. If we were half-asleep, and even if the other was asleep, the offender would say "sorry" after each one.

I'm in the hospital the day after they finally got the bleeding stopped. It was about three in the morning. I'm alone in my room, on my side with my back to the door, looking out the window at the George Washington Bridge. I was lonely, missing Rose, Louie and home, when I was overcome with the urge. Hell, I was alone, so I let it rip…with gusto. Man, that was a fart for the ages. I think my hospital gown had been turned to confetti as a result. And just because I was lonely, I said out loud, "Sorry." Immediately I heard a female voice behind me say, "Don't worry, it happens all the time." I turned and there she was, a nurse working on my IV bag! I hadn't heard her come in. I just wanted to die at that moment. I couldn't bury myself into the mattress deep enough, I was beyond embarrassed. Worst part of all? The nurse was pretty. When I told Rose, we laughed so hard that tears were streaming down both of our faces. When I finally got home, and we returned to our routine, we would laugh after every toot and consequent, "I'm sorry."

We both needed it. Funny what a fart can do, given the right situation.

69

From the moment I was told I would need a transplant I had a problem: *What was going to happen to my heart?* From the beginning I always assumed it should be returned to me, its rightful owner. I considered my heart to be a close friend, and here, even then, it was doing its best to keep me alive long enough for me to get its battlefield replacement. The idea of my heart being thrown onto a medical waste pile seemed to me to be the height of disrespect. So, once I'd established a rapport with my doctor and she understood the relationship I had with my heart, I told her that I wanted to take my heart home with me along with the new one. She didn't think the hospital would allow it. I was told that after its removal from my body the hospital took the position that I didn't own it anymore. Why not? It's mine! But that's not how they think of it. Well, I counter-argued, if the DNA in that heart proved I was guilty of a crime, I bet it would be mine *then*, right? It didn't matter. Logical arguments were not going to win that one. But I kept imploring her to help me get it, and she kept fighting for me. I love that doctor.

It was a serious issue to me. That heart and I had been through hell and back together, and I wasn't going to abandon my friend. It reached a point where she told me she was going to present my wishes to the board transplant board, which was to meet the night before our next appointment.

I came in for my appointment and met the male nurse who worked with my doctor. He was the first or second person I'd meet when we first went to that office, and he was an absolute Godsend. He made the journey easier than it might have been. He knew all about my desire to get my heart back and knew how the fight for it was going. So, just before I went in to see the doctor, he pulled me over and said these exact, life-changing words: "Tell them you want it for religious reasons." Genius! Of course, it was obvious, but it was he who thought of it.

Rose and I went into the exam room. My doctor was there with her head a little down and wearing a long expression on her face. She told me that she had met with the board and even though she prosecuted my wishes vigorously, they had voted no. She was sorry, she said, and I believed her. But I knew that what I had just been told by the nurse was surefire. Without missing a beat, I repeated exactly what I'd been told to say. As soon as I finished my statement, she dropped her forehead into the palm of her hand and let out the smallest groan. I knew at that moment I would get my heart. The nurse was right, they'd be too afraid of the lawsuit. I never would have sued, but they didn't know that. We live in a ridiculously litigious society. I knew they would never risk a lawsuit that was based on religious grounds. Thank you, Buddy!

It wasn't long after that when I was told I would be able to keep my heart. I hope I didn't cause my doctor any heat, but I knew she was glad I was going to keep it, too. She really understood.

Keeping my heart, however, was just the tip of a bigger iceberg. I was mourning the coming loss of my friend, and just as importantly the connection, the actual connection I'd been able to make between myself and my heart. That connection had kept me alive. It was no small thing. I remember when speaking with my doctor about my feelings of losing this friend, she had put her hand on my arm, looked me in the eye and with a small smile said, "Now you can make a new friend." The fact that she understood just how much it meant to me helped buoy my spirits, but, just as I had feared, it would not be possible, certainly not to the extent it had been with my own heart, to make friends with the new one. You see, when you get a new heart, they have to cut the nerve between the brain and your heart. Nerves don't grow back. That very real line of communication I had with my heart would be impossible with the new one. I've tried to make friends with this heart, but I can't reach it and it can't reach me. How can we become friends when we have no means of communication? But to whatever extent it's possible, we get along all right. And, wouldn't you know it? As time went on we did develop a friendship.

My asking for and being given permission to go home with both hearts had made me a minor celebrity at Columbia Presbyterian. Doctors would come into my room to work on me, realize who I was, and say, "It's you!" or, "So *you're* the one!"

After the transplant, Rose was made to sign a stack of papers an inch thick. It took her 40 minutes to complete the task. And there it was, in a little plastic container filled with alcohol and secured with a plastic lid. I became the first person in the history of Columbia to go home with both of their hearts and, to my knowledge, I must be one of the few people ever to hold his own heart in his hands, as I had to do when I transferred it to a more permanent sealed glass jar.

The only person who has seen my heart is Rose; I didn't get it for show-and-tell. I keep it in my office in one of my file cabinets. If I die first, it gets buried with me. If Rose dies first, it goes with her.

I'm the only guy I know who has literally given his heart to his wife.

70

From my very first hospital stay at North Shore I felt that I had to control the situation to whatever extent that I could. In every other time I had been in a hospital, from the first terrifying night at St. Francis till the last time when I was seventeen at LIJ, I had felt helpless and unable to control anything. I decided that first day at North Shore that would not be the case this time, or any other time, in my life again. So, I took control.

Doctors, nurses, techs, whomever, will come into your room, pick up your chart, and then announce they are there to do this or that to you and then proceed. It amazed me how many people who I had never seen before and would never see again paraded in and out of my rooms on my many stays. It was dizzying.

I started by asking who they were, why were they there, and then remind them to make sure my privacy and dignity were preserved. But most of all, I was always hyper-polite and would profusely thank anyone who did anything to and for me. I quickly gained a reputation as a patient who was a pleasure to be with. Now, isn't that going to help me more? They all liked me, wanted to help me, and they never got any grief from me. How could that be bad for me?

Three instances stand out from the rest. During my first hospitalization at North Shore, a tall, African American, straight-backed nurse strode into my room. Her expression was stern, but not angry. If I had to guess, I'd say she was ex-military. Where else do you learn the posture and precision that defined her? She was, in the best sense of the word, a handsome woman.

She went to my bed, picked up my chart and, without really looking at me, said, "I'm here to check on your groin." She was referring to the puncture site of my catheterization, which was next to the twins and their big brother. In other words, a perfect stranger was about to lift my gown and look at my most intimate parts. I asked her what her name was. She was a little startled by this but then told me. Then I asked her to please preserve my dignity. Still maintaining her officious bearing, she said, almost mechanically, "Don't worry; I've done this many times." I looked at her, she returned my gaze, and I asked, "Okay, can I inspect *your* groin?" She snapped straight up, furrowed her brow, and started thinking. After a few moments her entire demeanor changed; everything, her body language and the expression on her face just suddenly softened. *She got it.* She looked at me and said softly, "I'm here to look at your groin. Would that be okay?" Yes, it would, I responded, whereupon she gently lifted my gown, being extremely careful not to expose me more than necessary. When done, she put my gown down again gently. I LOVED this nurse! What a great woman! She *listened* to me, understood, and responded properly. We passed a few pleas-antries, and she left with both of us smiling.

The next incident also happened at North Shore. It was early, and the nurses were making their morning rounds. In walked a very pretty young nurse. Before I could ask her name, she asked me, "Have you moved your bowels today?" I looked at her with a smile and asked back, "Have you moved *your* bowels, today?" She got it instantly, and after a slight hesitation said, while laughing, "Well, yes I did." That became our little joke, and every morning she would walk in telling me first about her bowel movements of the day.

The third incident happened at North Shore, as well. I was in the bathroom and had just finished washing-up when a doctor, one of my doctors, knocked on the door. I told him to wait a minute. I was drying myself, no water was running, so he had no idea of what I was doing in there. He knocked again, and I said I'd be right out. Then he did the inexcusable. He walked into the bathroom. I was outraged. *How dare he!* Hey, you stupid moron, *you* work for *me*. I told him to get lost and when my cardiologist came in I told him what happened. I also told him to tell the other doctor he was fired, and I never wanted to see his face again and that he'd better not bill me for that morning visit. He didn't bill me and I never saw him again. Sometimes doctors forget who works for whom.

The point is you have to be your own advocate, then and there. Your family can't do it because they're not in the room when stuff happens. But you are, so it's up to you. You have to fight for your privacy and dignity. After a short while every doctor knew they had to be sure there were no gaps in the privacy curtain when they examined me. They knew they would have to explain what they were going to do, in detail, before they did it. And I was always polite to the max, and all the doctors and nurses enjoyed being with me.

If I ran a medical school, I'd make each first-year class get in hospital gowns—male and female—and walk the halls of the school with no underwear and with the non-slip socks they make you put on your feet. I'd make them stay in hospital beds for a week and have the second-year class examine them, make them see themselves as the patient does: half-naked and from a position that takes your power away. I'd make them use bedpans. I'd make them have blood draws in the morning. I'd make them experience—just for one week—what restricted water and salt intake is like. The list is almost endless.

I don't blame doctors. I love doctors, and I can easily understand their desire for a degree of detachment from their patients, so they can cope. I understand it, but at the same time I don't care. That's not my concern. *I'm their concern.* I think doctors should be more connected to the experience the patients have. I think if they are going to order a lifestyle change, they should at least have some understanding of what they are asking for, how difficult it could be, and offer first-hand strategies of how to do it and cope with it.

Imagine if doctors had to restrict their water for a week, let alone almost a full year. Don't you think they'd then have suggestions on how to do it? Don't you think they could be genuinely sympathetic and supportive?

So, the students would see one another nude. They want to see me nude, and you nude. They should have a comprehension of what that is like. After school, they will be seeing countless patients nude; touching their genitals, their breasts, putting a finger into their anus even if this was the first time they were meeting that patient, or even if it's the only time. They should understand from a first-person point of view at least a little of what the patients must endure. They should understand first-hand what the lack of dignity and the embarrassment feels like. It could only make them better doctors and better support systems for their patients. It just might make them seek ways of dealing with patients that provide a bit more dignity and a little less embarrassment. It might even knock some arrogance out of those that could use it.

Well, that's how I'd do it if I ran a medical school. In the meantime, make sure you are your own best advocate. And make sure you are kind, polite and gentle and *thank everyone* who comes in your room to do something for you—house cleaning, the phlebotomists who draw your blood, every single tech, nurse and doctor who walks into your room, you thank them! A lot! Who knows, it might even save your life.

71

It's March of 2001 and I'm really running out of steam. By the middle of the month I'm having doubts about being able to get the heart in time. I started getting the final details of my affairs in order. I made a package of my personal effects for Mark and made a few phone calls. I wasn't sure what the actual mechanism of my death would be. Would it be sudden, or would I die in a bed, gasping for breath until there was no longer enough oxygen in my system to support life? Both were possible. I called Chet and Larry and, without saying good-bye outright, they both knew what the call was about. Larry still refers to it to this day; Chet doesn't like to mention it.

I couldn't see it, but by this time I had lost all color. I've been told my face had become ashen. My lips were smaller and had lost all color, too. The lack of circulation also meant that I was always cold, couldn't eat too much, and my favorite muscle was getting so little circulation that I had to hunt for it to go to the bathroom; it was now playing turtle with me.

I could barely move; it took me forever to walk down my

hallway. But I still wouldn't stay in. I still went to the market most days, but even that was getting to be close to impossible. Joe said that walking with me was like being with George Burns walking through a foot of molasses. Larry tells me how painful it was for him to watch me walk up six steps, how I had to rest after each one. It was bad, and I knew it as did Rose and all my friends. There were a couple of times when I was out of the house when I thought I'd be dead in moments. Once, at my therapist's, I excused myself when the session had just begun because I thought I'd be lucky to have even a couple of minutes. I didn't want to die in his office, so as a courtesy to him I slowly made my way to my car and collapsed inside. I really didn't think I'd get out of that car, but it was a busy lot and I thought if something did happen, my body would be discovered soon enough. When I did finally get home all I could do was sleep, which was pretty much all I did at this point.

Even talking on the phone was too much, and after just a few sentences I'd be out of breath, have to hang-up and recover from the very short conversation. At night, Rose and I faced my position head-on. She knew how bad it was, and I would tell her it would be all right, thanked her for loving me, and to get on with her life after the dust settled.

There was a transplant group that met once a week in an old mansion in Manhasset. I had joined it a few months earlier. On March 26th, even as weak as I was, I was going to go to the meeting. After the meeting, I was supposed to go to a friend of Rose's, Claire, who held a Catholic Catechism class in her home. Apparently, the children who had been praying for me this whole time wanted to meet me.

They weren't the only ones praying for me. My brother's then girlfriend, a girl from Ireland, had a brother who was a priest. I was told his congregation prayed for me every week, as did a church in Port Jefferson, Long Island. But it was more than that. Because of the nature of my marketing business, I had groups and people praying for me all over the United States, along with the above-mentioned church in Ireland and a church in Italy, as well. I guess you could say that prayer-wise, I was covered.

I went to the mid-afternoon support group meeting. When I got out, I was wiped. It had snowed the day before, not too much, but I remember looking at the snow patches around me while I called Rose. I was leaning on the roof of my car as we spoke. I remember telling her I didn't think I had much time left. We had discussed this, and by this date we both agreed that in our opinions I had a week or two left—at most.

But I told Rose I still planned to see the children at Claire's Catechism class. I hung up and drove the 20 minutes to her house. I don't know what it was, but there was something compelling me to see them in spite of the way I felt.

Claire's home was neat and tidy and filled with children. I counted seven, including her daughter. I sat at the table they were using for their lessons and had a Coke with them. I was so out of it I really can't recall much of what we did or spoke about, but I do remember the feelings I got from those children were all positive.

Then Claire had us all join hands and we all recited the Lord's Prayer together. It was about half-way through the prayer when I felt something. It was almost like the chorus, except it was silent. But I got a jolt or a charge or *something*. I just can't put my finger on it, but I knew I had received another message. I couldn't interpret it, but I did receive it. After that, we all posed for a picture; me in the center with the kids all around me. I cherish that photo and have it framed in my office. In it you'll notice my hair was mostly dark brown with a little bit of silver peeking through.

I made it home and Rose wasn't there. She had been teaching at a local college. She worked night and day, and even after working from 8:00 a.m. to 7 or 8 p.m., she still brought an hour or two of work home with her each night. It was about 9:00 at night when my phone rang. I looked at the caller ID and saw it was Columbia making, I thought, another fund-raising call. We'd been told "the call," the one that said you had an organ, usually came around 3:00 in the morning. When I saw the caller ID, I almost didn't answer because I thought it was Columbia asking for a donation. They did this frequently enough and at about that time of the evening. I assumed that's what the call would be about. But, I figured, they were also trying to save my life, and so what if we made another donation? I answered the phone.

"Hello," I said in a bored voice.

"Hello, this is (sorry, I forgot her name) at Columbia Presbyterian."

"Yes," I answered in my still bored voice.

"Is this Steven Taibbi?"

"Yes, it is," I answered, still thinking this was a fundraising call.

"Are you sitting down?"

I was, but now I shot to my feet. "Is this *the call?*" I asked, with my heart in my throat.

"Yes, Steven, this is the call."

The rest of the conversation was a blur. But she told me we didn't have to rush because the heart was local. What she was really telling me was that the donor was close to Columbia, which would allow them to be able to wait until all the recipients were where they needed to be before they would proceed with the retrieval of those precious organs. I was instructed not to drive myself to the hospital, (yeah, right) and a couple of other things I can't really remember.

But I do remember my reaction to the words, "Yes, Steven, this is the call."

Imagine that a bucket crane—those cranes with the giant clamshell-like tongs that can scoop huge amounts of dirt with each pass—was above your head. And imagine that bucket was filled with every single emotion you have ever experienced in your entire life and that it opened above your head and all those emotions hit you all at once with great force. That's as good as I'll ever be able to explain it, but I think it's pretty accurate as to how it felt. No wonder they wanted you sitting, because I did fall back into my seat.

Those were the days when people wore beepers. I'd been given a beeper in case I wasn't home at the time of "the call." Rose wore one because she needed to be connected with her job. We'd worked it out that if I got the call while she wasn't home, I'd put "911" into her beeper. And that's what I did as soon as I got off the phone with Columbia.

A few moments later, Rose calls back in a panic. She was in her car, about 15 minutes from home when she got the 911. You have to love Rose and her powers of denial. Her first words to me were, "Are you kidding?" I couldn't help myself and answered her, "Yes, Honey, I'm just kidding." Of course, we both knew I wasn't kidding, and I just had to wait for her to come home.

In the meantime, one of the instructions I was given was not to call my friends in case it was a false alarm, which happens more often than you would think. So, when I got off the phone with Rose, I started to call my friends to tell them the news.

72

In the back of my mind I always knew I'd get the heart in time, even if I had my moments of doubt. But that phone call did something to me; it drove me even deeper into my Zen zone. I became unbelievably calm, almost in a dream state. Rose came home nearly in a panic. She would deny that, so I'll re-phase what I just wrote: Rose came home and acted as if she had just finished drinking 4,723 cups of coffee. Espresso. We had a go-bag ready for both of us, and we packed them and Louie into Rose's car and headed out...with me driving. Rose had called Michael and we were to meet him and his girlfriend at Columbia in front of the Milstein Building where we would hand Louie off to their care for the duration of my hospital stay.

Rose was frantic in the house for us to get on our way. I explained we had plenty of time; we were told to be there by 11:30 p.m. We didn't have to rush. If ever I wanted to drive a car, this was the time I wanted to the most. The hospital didn't want the patients to drive because they thought they'd be too excited to drive safely. Me? I knew this would be the last time I'd drive for weeks, if not forever, and I really wanted to enjoy it.

One might assume that under such circumstances I would drive with a "lead foot," but I didn't; I drove quite the opposite. The serenity I felt inside was being expressed by my right foot. It was driving Rose nuts who, for the first time since I'd known her, was asking me to drive faster. But we had time, I told her, and continued to enjoy myself by driving serenely, much to her exasperation.

There was also another factor that was to cause Rose much distress on our way to the hospital. Literally minutes before I received the phone call, I had taken my latest dose of Lasix, the diuretic. It wasn't long into the drive that the medicine took effect. I had to go, and I had to go *now*. I pulled over to a nearby train station that was on a fairly wooded lot, disappeared behind the trees, and came back much relieved. We resumed our journey. Shortly later I had to stop at a gas station but not to fill up. Between my driving speed and the second stop, I thought Rose's head was going to explode. And then, a little later, I had to stop for the third time. Rose was almost apoplectic. That was pretty funny to me, but Rose failed to see the humor in it, which was even funnier.

When we arrived at Milstein, Michael and his girlfriend were already there. I said my goodbyes to Louie, handed him off, and Michael's girlfriend left to drop Louie off at their mid-town apartment and then came back. We went to the location I had been directed to during the phone call and waited. I was fine with that. I knew the hospital knew what it was doing. After not too long a while we were met by a young woman who was as efficient as she was friendly. I was taken to a hospital room where I was given some medications that included a mild sedative. I was so calm, and deep in my zone, I never felt the effects of it.

A little while later we were taken to the holding room that was outside of three operating rooms. A young anesthesiologist, tall with curly blondish hair and who had a British accent, came out to meet me and answer any questions I might have. I liked him instantly.

I gave him my heart CD and told him I wanted it played during the operation. He took it and told me they had CD players with headphones, I could listen to it. No, I explained, I wanted the whole room to hear the CD; it was important to me. He then told me that only one of the three rooms had a stereo in it and he couldn't guarantee I would get that room, but he would be sure to play it if I did. I also told him I didn't want them to do anything to me until I was knocked out. Being into the zone I was already calm, but after speaking with him I was even more so.

Here's what could have happened: They could open me up, find out the new heart was no good, close me, and I'd wait again. They could open me up, plant the new heart, and it could reject immediately right there on the table, and with no other working heart around I'd die. I could just die on the table for the simple fact that sometimes the operation itself, any operation, can kill you. Or—and this was the most likely outcome of all—I'd get my new heart and along with it an extension on my expiration date.

After a short wait he came for me and told me they were ready. It was now about 3:00 a.m. I had requested that I be allowed to walk into the room, rather than to be wheeled in on a gurney, and he had agreed. So, we slowly walked toward the operating room, by good fortune the one with a stereo, and when we got to the doorway, I just stopped and soaked the room in. It was a beehive of activity. Just like many other times, I was greeted with the tinkle of surgical instruments being prepared, mixed with the hushed tones of everyone inside, with those who spoke quickly while they scurried to prepare for my change of heart. As I looked around, something dawned on me that was obvious, but had never occurred to me before. And for a reason I can't explain, it was important to me. When I was a kid and watched the "B" space movies of the fifties, or saw operating rooms or other control rooms depicted on TV, it always seemed to me that the rooms were special in that it appeared that the equipment in those rooms was somehow built-in, an inextricable part of the very walls and floors that made up the space. I turned to the doctor and said, "It's just a room with equipment in it." The doctor, who had a permanent small smile on his face, slowly looked around the room, and then at me, and said, "Yes, you're right. It's just a room with equipment in it." At that moment I was positive he could read my mind because I'm certain he understood my meaning. To this day, I can't express to you how important that small exchange was, and is, to me.

He directed me to the table, which I climbed onto by myself, (again, he was respecting my wishes) and immediately they started to strap me down. They had to do this as OR tables are very narrow to allow doctors to stand as close as possible to their work. Moments later a nurse came over to start an A-line. Before she could finish telling me what she was going to do, the doctor put his hand on her arm and gently said, "We're not going to do anything until Mr. Taibbi is asleep." Again, he was keeping his word. I love, *love*, this doctor.

They had put an IV access line in when I was in the first waiting room. The doctor now held the port in the IV line coming out of my right arm. He had already put a needle in the port and gently asked me, "Do you have any other questions?" I told him I didn't.

"Are you ready?"

"Yes," I said.

As he pushed the plunger in, I turned my head and looked at the ceiling lights above me. That's all I remember, because Versed turns you off like a light switch. One moment I was there, and the next I was gone. Snap! Just like that.

After the operation, a doctor asked my brother if they could keep my heart CD. He said they could. I couldn't think of a better place for it.

73

It seems that the more often they knock me out, the more I want to stay below the waves of the comforting sea. But after a certain time, they have to wake you, and that was how it was with me. I just didn't want to come back, but the nurse was insistent; reluctantly I did. I was still on a ventilator, a machine with a tube that goes down your throat and helps you to breath. This is the machine that is commonly mislabeled "life-support" by everyone, especially the media.

So back I came, heavily drugged with pain killers and the inability to open my eyes for more than a few seconds at a time; my eyelids were simply too heavy. But the moment I came back I was aware of something that I would have bet everything I owned on, something I was sure about that entire year, that when I woke Rose would be holding my hand. And she was. I could feel the soft skin of her hand pressed into mine. I have to say in spite of being drugged and in an enormous amount of pain, it made me smile inside.

The pain *was* enormous. The most pain I ever experienced

from an operation in my life. Later, the surgeon who performed the transplant told me that I had so many *adhesions*, a form of internal scar tissue, from my two previous open-heart surgeries that he had to "hack and saw" his way through it. That explained the pain.

When I woke, not including the intubation tube in my throat, I had an additional 13 tubes and wires coming out of me. But I rallied quickly, and the intubation tube was removed in just a few hours, which was earlier than it usually is. There are too many stories of that time in critical care, but I think it's enough to know that I did well there. I was moved to a step-down room after only two or three days. But I was far from recovered and still in enormous pain.

In spite of the pain, shortly after I woke I knew I was better. I could barely move, barely keep my eyes open, but I could feel the difference; I wasn't cold, and my hands and feet were warmer than they'd been for a long time. I could *feel* the improved circulation. Rose said my face and lips had color again.

A lot happens to a patient in a hospital after a heart transplant. In the beginning, some tube or wire or IV line is removed every day, some painfully, some with great relief. In the step-down room I still had two or three IV's going through both hands. That made sleep an interesting proposition. You had to teach yourself that if you want to roll to the left, and then to the right, you must first roll onto your back and then roll in the other direction, so as not to get tangled in the IV lines.

A couple of things stand out from those 11 days at Columbia. First, there were nights where the pain was enormous, all-encompassing, times when I was literally writhing, clutching my chest and incapable of any voluntary movements whatsoever. They had to be careful about the amount of painkillers they could administer even though those pesky adhesions that had been "hacked and sawed" through were exacting their revenge on me in spades. I had a roommate, and he had the window bed. At night, I scared him a couple of times when I was in those instances of uncontrollable pain.

I was also on huge doses of prednisone, a steroid. It turns you into a crazy person, giving you astoundingly wild swings in your emotional state. One moment, you are laughing uncontrollably and the next you're crying like a baby. Every time my doctor walked into the room, I was so grateful that I'd just start crying. I'm still on prednisone, but only five milligrams, which is a pretty good indication of just how massive the beginning doses were. Nevertheless—and I've spoken with other transplants about this—TV commercials can make us cry. Forget about emotional movies!

There was also something else that many of us experienced while in our transition at Columbia; we felt safe there. If anything, God forbid, was to happen, we knew we were in the best possible place and could get immediate and expert care. After the event of the transplant, I *wanted* to be at Columbia. Also, Columbia is a remarkably good hospital that does more than provide world-class care. In all my stays and visits there, I only ran into one bad nurse and that was for only one night. Everyone, from the parking attendants all the way up, were always looking to see if there was a way they could be helpful to you. I'll give two examples.

When my roommate was discharged before me, his bed had to be sterilized. A woman in her thirties came in. She barely spoke English and I guessed she was Hispanic. She set to the task. There wasn't a surface of the bed frame she didn't wash down, including *under* the bed. She washed that bed as if the next person who was to occupy it was going to be her own child. Who knows, she might have saved a life.

Then there was the night custodian. He was a tall, thin African-American man, and he cleaned the hall floors with one of those giant floor dusters. No biggie? It was to me. I looked forward to him making his rounds. He came by late when most of the patients were well asleep, but I still had my night-owl ways. What made him special was that he always whistled while he worked. Not loudly, but at the same time, happily. He never stopped, never seemed down, always did his work well, and always seemed happy to do it. He'll never know it, but I looked forward to hearing his joyful whistling. The sound and sight of him made me feel safe, and that all was right with the world.

At the same time, I wondered about my donor: Who was he, how had he died, how was his family doing? I felt such gratitude towards him and his family that it's impossible to put it into words. How could I thank him? Thank all the donors that make transplantation possible and not just a wish? *Well*, I thought, *you're already a professional public speaker in marketing*, and I vowed then that I would use my skills as a speaker to be a voice for donation, both as a thank you and to raise public awareness.

In about a week they were introducing me to the starting cocktail of anti-rejection drugs I'd be on for the rest of my life and getting me ready to go home. I wanted to go home because it was my mother's eightieth birthday, while at the same time I never wanted to leave. But finally, on April 7th, one day after my mother's birthday and eleven days after admission, I was discharged and sent on my way with a new lease on life, someone else's heart in my chest, and to start my new life as a heart transplant.

74

When we got home, Louie was, of course, crazy-happy to see me. Being I wasn't allowed to lift anything over ten pounds, Rose picked him up and gave him to me. But as soon as Louie got close to my chest he freaked! He heard the new heartbeat and didn't know what to make of such a change and started to squirm violently in my arms. Rose had to take him back. He didn't know how to react. He knew it was me, but what was the deal with that heartbeat? I'm positive he knew the heart wasn't mine, but how did it get there? he must have wondered. I'm fairly sure dogs aren't taught about heart transplants in obedience school, so he was clueless. In about a week, he got used to the new sound in my chest and became his old self with me and continued to be my shadow.

I hadn't showered since before the transplant and it would be a couple of weeks after I arrived home before I would finally be allowed. The doctors were afraid of the bandages getting wet and thus causing infection. About the eighth day after surgery, I couldn't stand myself any longer and stuck my head under the faucet of the sink in my room, washed my hair, and gave myself a sponge-bath to the extent possible, considering all the new holes in me that couldn't get wet. It did make me feel great, but you can imagine how much I was looking forward to taking a real shower.

When I got home, I got my first good look at myself in a full-length mirror. I not only felt like I'd been hit by a truck, I looked like it too. My entire chest from just below the clavicles to a few inches below my naval was an angry, deep, black, purple and blue, with a touch of yellow and light orange here and there. I have to admit, I was startled by the sight of myself. But finally, it was time for me to take my first shower. I remember it like it was yesterday. I made sure the water was the perfect temperature. When satisfied, I stepped in, facing the shower as I did in anticipation of enjoying the best shower of my life. When the water hit my chest I almost screamed. It felt like small ball peen hammers were being thrown at my chest by Thor himself! I quickly turned around and made the shower as short as possible while exposing my fragile chest to the pounding water as little as possible. Afterward, while I felt refreshed and clean for the first time in weeks, I also had to recover from the shower itself. It hurt for more than an hour. Drying myself became its own adventure. After that, the last thing I wanted to do was take a shower. Every heart transplant I've spoken with about this had the same experience. All of us had been deeply disappointed, as well.

This was my first real lesson, the one that taught me it's not easy to be a transplant. That has held true for every single day since I received this wonderful gift.

75

Not long after I came home, about six weeks or so, two events happened that helped shape my new transplant life. The first event was the wedding of one of Rose's cousins. This was going to be the first time since the surgery that the bulk of Rose's family would see me. "Bulk" is the correct word, as there had to be at least 118,753 of Rose's immediate family in attendance. That might be a slight exaggeration, but if you'd been in my shoes that day I'd bet you'd agree that number was at least in the ballpark.

They all wanted to speak with me; they all had a million questions. They'd open the conversation with, "You look good" and then launch into their questions. Look, all those people kept me in their prayers, and that's no small thing in my book, and they all wished me well. But after you've had the exact same conversation a couple of hundred times in a row, it just gets wearing. So, the first quick answer I came up with, after I was told I looked good was, "It was my heart, not my face," a line I still use. Then, and only because I was worn out by the same repeating conversation, I started to answer all the questions with, "I'm still not dead." Again, a line I still use.

Uncomfortably, whenever we went out, I became the center of all conversation, as everyone wanted to know what it was like to have a heart transplant. Often, I couldn't stand it. I just wanted to be normal. All my life–a lifetime of heart trouble–I'd made it a point that my heart issues were as far in the background as possible. People never spoke to me about my heart. But now it was all people would speak to me about. It's understandable. They'd spent that year waiting with me, in one way or another, and they were happy that when I was done walking that 50/50 line I'd fallen onto the side of life. I even had to ask a friend of mine to stop introducing me as a guy who just had a heart transplant. He certainly meant well, but I was being branded for the first time in my life as a heart patient. Unfortunately for me, the very nature of being a transplant, and all the issues one brings in tow as such, branded me as a heart patient. After a lifetime of being able to keep my heart problems in the distance, they were now too much in the forefront. It is just part of the price a transplant has to pay to be "still not dead." That line became a promise between Rose and me. I love to joke, and I'm convinced that humor is a big factor in my survival thus far. I've always told Rose that I hope my last words are the funniest joke I've ever told. Who knows, it probably won't happen. But this, I assure you, will happen: I've asked Rose, and she has promised me, that when I die my headstone will read, "*Now* I'm dead." At the very least it might bring a smile to someone who is at the cemetery and could use a lift of spirit. No matter, having that phrase on my stone is now very important to me.

Six weeks after transplant, my desire to be a speaker on the cause of transplantation came true. Rose's hospital was doing an event on transplantation, and since everyone in the hospital knew Rose and our circumstances, I was asked if I'd like to speak at that event, which, of course, I would. I was supposed to have 15 minutes, but there were several politicians there and they all ran long; what a surprise. By the time my turn came I was told I had three minutes and three minutes only. From both my television and speaking careers I have a very good internal clock. I spoke for two minutes and fifty-eight seconds. Rose kept time but didn't signal me, and there was barely a dry eye in the house. Also in attendance were a couple of people from the New York Organ Donor Network, or NYODN, (now known as Live On New York) the Organ Procurement Organization (OPO) that I received my heart through. Afterwards, they wanted to know if I'd like to speak for them sometimes, and, of course, I said yes. That little presentation was about to set a course for me that would last for fourteen years.

One last thing about that time. The day I went into the hospital for the transplant, as I said earlier, I'd taken a group picture that afternoon with those kids. In it, my hair was mostly dark-brown with some grey. We'd taken some pictures of me and my family the day after I got out at my mother's eightieth birthday, and more were taken of me at the aforementioned wedding.

Pictures don't lie. Sometime between the transplant and when I was released, my hair had become almost entirely silver. None of us noticed it until we saw the pictures.

76

I t isn't easy to be a transplant, but it's nothing one should be complaining about, either. And there are those that do. God gives you this great gift, you're still alive and mostly functional, and to complain about how tough it can be seems to me to be ungrateful. Hey, you complainers! *You're still not dead!* Go and smell the roses.

The first year is the hardest. They must figure out the medicine cocktail that is right for you, you have to go to the hospital starting at every two weeks, to every three, and then every month, and finally every three months. Every three months is forever. In the beginning, those visits also equate to biopsies, an invasive procedure where they go through a vein in your neck, send a catheter down to measure pressures in your lungs and then go into your new organ to take a piece of your heart (yes, they have the Janis Joplin song in the room!) and check to see if you're rejecting or not.

The drugs can be murder. For some, there is absolutely no issue with them. For others, like me, it's a nightmare where the side effects can make life unpleasant, to say the least. But you're still not dead, and if this is the price I and others have to pay, then so be it. Really, it's cheap enough and I'm more than willing to pay it to still be here.

I'd been speaking, mostly at venues I'd found on my own and some for NYODN, when NYODN invited me to a "speakers training" they were hosting that was being given by Transplant Speakers International, Inc. I went and at the end of the day they asked me to join. At my first TSI meeting I was also told I was on the board as well.

TSI was founded by Columbia Pres heart transplants Peter Radigan and Frank Bodino, and Ed Masol and Donald Arthur (now both deceased), along with Ed's wife, Pat Meldin, who was a donor family member, and Jack and Arlene Locicero, whose daughter, Amy, was the last victim of the Long Island Railroad massacre in 1993. Amy was an organ donor. They all recognized the need for greater awareness about organ and tissue donation. They had the idea they could help achieve that goal by teaching the volunteers of the various OPOs across the country to present their stories at speaking venues. Soon I was traveling all over the country, once or twice a month, giving trainings usually with Jack, or Dave Lively, whose son had also been a donor. I've been from New York to Hawaii, Texas to Minnesota, Massachusetts to Florida, and most places in between.

We had a program Jack and Arlene started called, "Sorrowful Joy" for the families of the donors. It was a support group to help those families who'd lost loved ones cope with dealing with the unique loss and the situation of that person also becoming a donor. I honestly can't tell you how many times I've heard a donor family member tell me that the donation was the only thing that made any sense of an otherwise senseless death. Donors, as I said before, by the very nature of the requirements necessary for organs to be usable, almost always died from a sudden trauma. The donations gave these families a great deal of peace.

I had a bad case of survivor's guilt. When I'd go on one of my training trips, which usually lasted two days, the donor stories about how loved ones died were almost unbearable. When I came home I often needed at least two days just to recover. In the beginning, survivor's guilt was eating me up, and when I made my presentation at the trainings it became apparent to one and all—especially me. But for some reason no one wanted to deal with the survivor guilt issue—not the doctors, nurses, or families, not even those at the OPOs. Frank and I shared a few stories between us about just that. It was incredible. Rather than deal with our guilt, we were often told by others we were ungrateful, something someone in my own family told me. We are *extremely* grateful. But we were also wracked with guilt. After all, we had all been ready to die if that was what was to be. We were *prepared*. Our donors, on the other hand, weren't; they had no idea they were going to die that day. Many of us would have gladly traded places with our donors because we were ready, and they weren't.

If we tried to express that guilt, however, whether it was to a doctor, nurse, family member or member of an OPO—no matter to whom—we were always, and I mean *always*, shut down. Again and again the response was, "They didn't die for you," or "They were going to die anyway!" They all seemed to think, okay, you got your organ, move on. But if you have half an ounce of compassion, it just isn't that simple.

Think of it this way: If a woman loses her breast to cancer and then, rightfully, mourns that loss and expresses it, no one says to her, "Well it was going to kill you" or "Well, you have another." *NO!* They sympathize with her, saying things like,

"That must be tough" or "I'm sorry you have to go through this," or "This must be difficult for you." No matter what they say, they don't shut her down with a platitude.

This really started to bug me. I went to Frank, our president, and by then I was vice-president, with an idea for another support group to address this very issue. Rose came up with the perfect name, Grateful Guilt. Frank approved, I designed it. Frank and I massaged it, and it became part of our program. Grateful Guilt and Sorrowful Joy both ran an hour before the start of training, populated by volunteers who wanted to attend the appropriate session. The response was startling. We recipients had all been shut down up to this point, but now our feelings of survivor's guilt were finally being acknowledged. many thought there must have been something wrong with *them*, they been shut down often. I saw a grown man fall onto his hands and knees, sobbing almost uncontrollably, when his feelings were finally allowed to come out. The OPOs were shocked at the reactions. Now they understood this was a real issue in the transplant population and started to treat it as such.

Lately, I've begun to hear that some others are trying to take credit for the program or the acknowledgement of these pent-up feelings. I'm here to tell you that we were the first; it was Transplant Speakers International, Inc. that brought this issue to the front and TSI were the first to do something about it.

And that's the truth.

77

So many times while sitting alone with Louie on my lap I would think about my potential donor. I would wonder who'd they'd be, how they would die, and if they were somehow more prepared to die than most who had no idea that a particular day would be their last. Often, I would wish I could time travel and take the hit for them because I was ready, and they were not; because I was the one near death and they were healthy with a whole life ahead of them. This, of course, was the start of my survivor's guilt and it would pain me, deeply, that I couldn't take that hit for them.

I know a little bit about my donor. I know he was ten years younger than me and he was a black male, which should put to rest the idea that race is a barrier to donation between any race and any other. Skin color is just that—a color—the outside color. Inside, we're all blue and red, and just like the Model T, our parts are interchangeable. I wrote the family a letter but I never heard back from them and if they don't want to respond, well, that's their right and I respect it. Completely. This is not uncommon; only 3% of donor families respond to letters.

Of course, I have no idea who he was, who his family is. When you write your letter, you send it to your OPO and they forward it for you. I will never be told where he lived or what his or his family's name is. The recipient isn't allowed to give any of that information about themselves, either. If, after they receive your letter and they wanted to meet you, they would have to indicate through the OPO, who then would pass that info to you. If both parties agreed to meet, it would then be arranged, and after that you'd be on your own.

I know almost nothing about my donor, but I can tell you the following about his wife, or next of kin. I know that they are generous and loving. Even if he always wanted to be a donor, the law, as it was then in New York state, would have allowed the family to deny it. The law has since been changed. But we know they said yes. I imagine he was married and the decision was left to the wife, but that's sheer conjecture on my part. I don't know if he was a donor, but when she was asked her response was something similar to, "Yes, he would have liked that."

Here she is, again, this part is my imagination, but it's true for any spouse that consents—she has just been told her husband —her lover, her friend, the father of her children, and a provider of the household—had just died and she has the *grace* to say yes, to see past her own tragedy and help to extend the lives of others.

I also imagine my donor was one who gave multiple organs. Here's how I imagine that: I received his heart, two people got his lungs, someone got his liver, one person got one kidney, and another person got the other along with his pancreas that they're no longer a Type I diabetic. Two other people received his corneas. The corneas are considered a tissue donation, and tissue donations are every bit as important as organ donations are. So, even though he died young, he saved the lives of eight people, and that is pretty good in my book. Yes, I believe giving someone back their sight is akin to saving a life. Well, that's what I imagine, and it happens often enough in the world of donation.

My donor and his family will forever be in my prayers. We set a place for him at the table the first holiday we had after my transplant, and on the holidays since. There will never be words adequate enough that can express my gratitude to my donor and his family and to *all* donors and their families. It is they who make transplantation possible. Without them, transplantation is just a wish.

While we're on the subject of transplantation, I'd just like to spend a few moments on brain death. The way the OPO's explain it and the way the press misreports it leaves most people with no real clue to what it is. This confusion causes vast amounts of people to decide *not* to become donors and leaves countless families with pain that can only be considered cruel. I'm sorry, but I'm about to be blunt.

Recently on national news was the story of a young child who died during a routine operation. The parents were told she had suffered brain death, yet as the press breathlessly reported, she was on *life support*. Brain death or not, the parents refused to take her off life support, refused to believe she had died because she was on *life support!* The parents suffered cruelly because in spite of the words *brain death*, the only thing they heard was *life support*.

So, let's get a few things straight: *Brain death is death*. Period. *Once the brain dies, you are dead*. End of subject. There is no coming back from brain death no matter what the machine your loved one is plugged into is mislabeled.

The bottom line is this: *We all die of brain death*. You had a heart attack? Well, you didn't die because you had a heart attack, you died because there no longer was a heart to pump blood and oxygen *to your brain*. You are alive after a fatal heart attack for as long as your brain can hold out without that circulation. Look, I had no heart at all once mine was taken out and until the new one was put in, sutured, and re-started. I didn't die because I was hooked up to a heart-lung machine that took over the functions of those two organs while I had no heart in me at all.

Here's another: A person is pulled from the water; no heartbeat and they aren't breathing. Yet if appropriate measures are taken in enough time they can come back because their brain hasn't died yet. Wait too long and they have brain damage from a lack of oxygen. A little bit after that, and they can't come back because the brain has died.

Police tell stories of a people crazed on drugs who have had their heart shot to pieces but continue to shoot their guns and even kill others for a couple of minutes.

So, understand, *brain death is death*.

But...but... but, the person is on life support! They're breathing! They're still warm! *They're on LIFE support!*

That's all true, but they are dead, they have passed, and they are never coming back. The confusion comes from the words *life support*. If you're not informed about these things it's easy to think, *well, why would they be on life support if they're dead?* The simple answer is they are not on life support; they are on a *ventilator*, a machine that takes over the function of the lungs when the lungs can no longer function on their own. There are times when the living is put on these machines for various medical reasons. I've been on them, and loosely I guess you could call that "life support," but really, it's still a ventilator, and can never be life support for the brain dead. Once you are brain dead, your heart and various other functions of the body can continue, but these are automatic responses. But they can't go on forever.

When the brain dies, so does animation, and necrosis sets in. From the moment my donor died, necrosis started, which is why there is such a time factor in transplantation. Wait an hour or two too long, and the organ will no longer be viable. Same happens to a brain-dead body on a vent. Ventilator or not, the body has started the process of returning to dust.

So, the next time you hear someone call it "life support" please correct them. Few things hurt me more than watching a family refuse to let go of a loved one who is no longer with us because they believe there is still a chance because that loved one is still on "life support."

And really, what could be crueler than that?

78

Earlier, I'd alluded to the fact that for my entire lifetime since I was five, I have lived in fear and shame, that I sabotaged relationships and parts of my career because of this fear, because of this certain knowledge that I was no good. It's been impossible to tell me that it's all in my head, that I'm wrong about this. Sorry, I *know*, somewhere inside of me, I'm no good. And because of it, I'm afraid. All of the time. Exceptions exist, but they are far and few between and don't last for more than hours.

Obviously, I've always been aware of this, knew that it kept me from a full and happy life, but—and this is no exaggeration —I couldn't do anything about it. I had no control over it whatsoever.

Also, certain things bothered me much more than it did anyone else I knew. The best example is the concept of unfairness. Whether it was something that was unfair to me, someone else, or even the government doing things that were unfair, unfairness infuriated me. This would trigger an outsized response, and infuriation would quickly turn to burning anger. This never caused me to become physical, except when I was a child and finally dealt with bullies. But, really, that was self-defense. I have never lashed out physically at anyone, no matter how furious I was since that last bully at school. So, while I knew there were things that would drive me nuts, I also knew I could control it, at least to a degree that mattered. Also, and I know this about myself, it's just not in my nature to want to hit people or want to harm them in any way. If anything, my anger would always ultimately turn inward, towards myself for being the way that I was. I could be depressed for days after I'd have an outburst of anger, which never escalated past yelling, but I always took it as another example that inside, I really was bad.

It's not like I didn't try to get help. When I was sixteen, I went to the school counselor who recommended me to a public child psychiatrist. At my first visit she questioned my use of a word she thought I'd used incorrectly, when I knew (and I was right) I hadn't. That started us on a bad note as far as I was concerned, but I looked past it and tried to get the help I knew I needed. But it turned out she was useless, and I quit her after just a few months.

Then one night, years later when I was in my late twenties or early thirties, I was on the phone with a dear friend of mine, Eileen. We were both watching *All That Jazz* from our respective homes when the open-heart surgery scene appeared. They had already opened the chest of the main character and were cranking his chest apart with rib spreaders. And then it happened. Something in me broke: a dam of pent-up feelings and denial that had, to that point, kept me completely emotionless about all my operations and pain. That dam that had made it possible for a doctor to cut into me without an anesthetic, and I wouldn't move or make a sound. But that scene did it, those rib spreaders did it, and the dam had finally been breached, and the next thing I know, I'm on the floor sobbing into the phone with Eileen while a lifetime of pain and fear flooded over me.

I found a therapist a friend recommended and had my first visit with her about two weeks later. She helped me tremendously, and after some years we finished. I was better, but that basic truth that somewhere deep I was bad and my feelings towards unfairness, persisted.

A few years ago, I decided I was tired of living in fear, that by hook or by crook, I was going to get to the bottom of this, so help me God. I'd been told that there were MSW's who specialized in those kinds of things, and I found Sarah Zimmerman, who it turns out is about as good as it gets.

She knew what the problem was within minutes of our first meeting. We've worked hard together to deal with it. I would say we're 90 percent or more done, and thankfully my life is vastly improved. I would say my anger is down by that same percentage. I haven't had an outburst in several years. We're getting down to the nub, and I finally was able to describe feelings I haven't been able to even identify until now.

It started when I was five, with the incident with the NO FOOD sign. That feeling of complete powerlessness, *that abandonment of all hope*, was the first time I "broke." But it was more than that. It was also the fact that my will never mattered; I'd have no say whatsoever in what was going to happen to me. Yes, my mother would tell me that I was going to be "Buck Rogers" with the anesthesia mask, but no one, *no one*, ever told me what was going to happen or asked if it was okay to operate on me, to cut me, to change the way I'd look forever. All I knew was that the next day, men in white outfits were going to come with a gurney to collect me. I'd have to smell that horrible ether and bear the monstrous headache that was guaranteed to follow, and that somewhere on my body I'd have pain and stitches, and I'd never look the same again.

When it came time for my first open heart, waking in an oxygen tent in such horrific pain was a complete shock. I had no idea that was what was going to happen, that I'd be split open and in agony for days and days. Till then, I'd had no idea it was even possible to be in that much pain.

It all made me feel invisible, inconsequential and worthless. My feelings didn't matter. I just had to surrender my body while I was forced to dissociate into my cave or on the back of my seagull.

Sarah finally put a name to what was wrong. I had Complex Trauma. Complex Trauma is most akin to PTSD, Post Traumatic Stress Syndrome. PTSD is the result of single-event trauma, whereas my trauma was reoccurring with new traumas even to this day. Like the little girl who lays awake at night wondering if her father would be coming into her room for a "special visit," I did the same wondering if tomorrow would be a "special visit" day for me.

Complex Trauma is layered like an onion, making it difficult to deal with from the clinical point of view, whereas single trauma PTSD can often be dealt with in months. Complex Trauma patients aren't violent because we tend to blame ourselves and turn our negative feelings inward, because we *know* it's all our fault.

Why had no one caught this before? Because even up to the *DSM-IV*, (the *Diagnostic and Statistical Manual of Mental Disorders*, Edition IV) the clinical manual that gives the diagnosis that was current when I met Sarah, Complex Trauma was not listed or described. As a result, most doctors and MSW's don't know what to look for or what to call it, it is often, and wrongly, called PTSD. Sarah, and those like her who recognize so-called

Complex Trauma, are anxious for it to be included in the *DSM*, but until it is, there will be many like me who, even though they are seeking help, won't get the proper treatment because the ailment is not described, nor is the appropriate therapy.

Well, I'm almost there in the battle to combat the Complex Trauma that's been with me since I was five. This might be the most difficult thing I've ever taken on. But I'm in a much greater sense of peace nowadays and that fear, that nagging fear is, for the most part, no longer there.

Without Sarah, I wouldn't have gotten this far, and I can't wait until I finally complete this particular journey. I'm lucky to have her walking next to me on this difficult path of my life.

79

There is an old Chinese saying, meant as a curse: "May you have an interesting life." Well, I've certainly had an "interesting life." But I wouldn't call it cursed. In fact, when I think about it, *blessed* would seem to be more appropriate. It hasn't been easy, but really, whose life is? In spite of living a life dominated with Complex Trauma, multiple instances of nearly dying, and a never-ending parade of hospital and doctor visits, I'm glad I have the life I have. I've been taught lessons at a very young age that most people don't learn until they're in their final years. I learned not to be afraid of death, but instead to embrace it, and this gave me the freedom to live a fairly unconventional life. For better or worse, I've lived life on my terms, working only for myself and unafraid to take risks. Truly, *not* taking risks in life is as scary to me as *taking* risks are to most people.

I had my first business at fourteen. Started my television business two weeks before I graduated college. I was a songwriter, partner in a small advertising agency, and had an aviation company for film and video. I've worked with presidents and top CEO's and the largest corporations in the world. I became a pilot and owned my own glider. I changed careers to a marketing business and now I'm back to my first love of being a photographer.

More importantly, I've been given life-changing lessons. Maybe the biggest is my perception of God, miracles, and my belief in Him.

I look at miracles in a different way than anyone else I know. A life suddenly being saved, a result that seemed impossible but happened despite the odds, heck, even moving a mountain, none of these are miracles to me, they're just parlor tricks.

This is what a miracle is to me: I needed a new heart and the right doctor to save my life. The miracle here is that through uncountable generations, the right people married the right people and the result produced my doctor where I needed her and when I needed her. The exact same thing applies to my donor. And, in extension, this applies to every single person who was a cog in the wheel of the miracle that saved me. Now, *that's* a miracle.

I also learned that I don't need a religion, or a church, to worship and love God. He is always around me, always with me. I don't need a special day of the week or a building to say "Hi" to stay in touch. I am always in touch with Him and He is always in touch with me.

I believe in an all-powerful God. There are no limits to His Grace or Might. It was this realization that made me stop going to church. The God I believe in can't be contained by one church or religion. The God I believe in won't send you to Hell if you belong to this religion instead of that one. But I have found that most people don't believe in an all-powerful God, even though they say they do, and I can prove it. I discovered the starkest example of this after my transplant when I became a speaker on donation. There are people, entire religious groups, who think you can't donate because if you do you won't be able to get into Heaven, that you have to be "whole" to get in. Forget about the fact that there is not a single major religion that doesn't agree with donation; these people refuse to believe otherwise. I've run into people like this in every major religion. Some entire churches and temples believe this way, even though their religions—as opposed to a particular church or temple—disagree with them.

So, let's look at this. The God these people believe in, the one who created the entire universe, won't let you into Heaven if you've donated your lungs or heart or anything else? He doesn't have the power to restore you? If someone loses a leg, is he called "Stumpy" when he or she gets to Heaven? What a small god (lower case "g" is deliberate) such a person believes in. Truth is, I think that to many, the concept of a truly all-powerful God scares the pants off them or is simply incomprehensible. No wonder many are terrified at the thought of their own mortality.

I stopped going to church after transplant because of this belief. For me, going to church would be telling God I don't think He is all powerful, and worse, it would be throwing the precious lesson He gave me, through his Grace, back into His face.

My family doesn't understand my feelings about this, and I think several of them assume my next stop is Hell. But if someone wants to go to church or temple, be involved to whatever degree they are in their religion, I say go for it! If that is what is right for you, if that's how you have your connection to God, I'm happy for you. These are just my thoughts about God and the lessons I've been given. Your lessons are most likely entirely different. My feelings on this subject pertain only to me.

Like me, you have to follow your own path and where it takes you.

Two final thoughts on donation. Doctors, nurses, medical professionals and reporters, please, I'm begging you, *please*, stop using the word *harvested* when speaking about donated organs and tissue. Corn is harvested. Wheat is harvested. Humans, *people*, are not. It's funny, but the donor families don't object to that word as much as recipients do. We find it grossly insulting to the families of the donors and deeply disrespectful. How about instead saying, "The organs were *recovered*," or "*you received the gift.*" Additionally, it's hard enough to get donors. Maybe if they didn't think they'd be harvested, there might be more of them. I'm begging you, show respect to the families and stop referring to donors as a crop or a commodity. Really, isn't that the least we should do?

And for those who have "religious" reasons, or any other, for not signing-up to be donors, I have a question for you: What do you think God would want us to do with organs and tissue after someone dies? Which do you think He would prefer after He gave the gift of your life to you? That we bury or burn them or pass them on and save other lives? Please, give it some thought.

So, that's my story. I hope you found it helpful and I thank you for spending your time with me.

Remember, the clock is ticking...for all of us. So...go out and live!

May you always be aware of the blessings that surround you.

EPILOGUE

I had pretty much finished this book more than two years ago. I figured it would be published in maybe three to six weeks from then. I was making the video trailer for *Grateful Guilt* on my 62nd birthday, April 26, 2015. We were almost done shooting the trailer when I had a massive heart attack. Thing is, being a heart transplant, I didn't know what had just happened because I didn't feel anything. When they transplant you, they obviously cut out your heart so they can replace it with the donor organ, and in doing so, cut the nerves to your heart – and nerves never grow back. So, I had no sensation of the heart attack, I just started shivering, it was pretty cold out, and I felt awful. My assistant on the shoot, Haydee Torres, noticed the change in me and came over. She looked at me hard and said, "I don't like the way you look". The show must go on, as the old adage says, and we finished the shoot. When I got home, I just went straight to bed, and in my bones, I knew something was wrong.

This happened on a Friday and on Monday we, Rose and I,

went into the city to see my doctor at Columbia. After a very brief exam, she told me in no uncertain terms that she was getting a bed for me at the hospital *right now* because she wanted me on telemetry. Telemetry is when they put electrodes on you, like those used for an EKG, with a small radio transmitter you carry on your person that sends the signals to a central nursing station on your floor so they can monitor you twenty-four hours a day.

We had known for quite a while that I had Transplant Coronary Artery Disease, something only heart transplants can get. It's a form of rejection. With TCAD, the arteries in your heart start to close down in much the same way they do with regular Coronary Artery Disease, except that instead of fat and plaque clogging the vessels, it's inflammation of the vessels doing the damage.

We already knew this process had started and I already had two stents to prove it. My doctor was doing everything she could to keep it at bay, but TCAD is unpredictable and it can advance suddenly. So, the next day it was back to the cath lab for three more stents followed by the news that this heart, too, was on the way out. Yet again, I had about a year to get another heart or die if I didn't.

So, once again the battle had started, and I was on my way to my fourth open heart operation, my second heart transplant and, what would be, my third heart.

There is just something about April 26th, isn't there?

ACKNOWLEDGMENTS

The author would like to thank those who lent a helping hand in making this book possible. Your moral and material support are appreciated more than you'll ever know: Debbi Honorof, Brian McKernan, Harriet Shrewood, Sarah Zimmerman and publishing consultants Carol Hoenig and Stephanie Larkin.

And a special thanks to Harry (himself a 20 year kidney transplant) and Maria Korines, owners of The Golden Coach Restaurant, along with Jeanne Fry, Cathy Busch-Pavlik and Andrew Vagenas where the majority of this book was written. Thanks for keeping the iced tea coming, guys! Last but not least, a special thanks to all the doctors, nurses, techs and hospital workers of all kinds who have successfully kept me past my expiration date especially Dr. Donna M, who has my everlasting gratitude.

ABOUT THE AUTHOR

Steven Taibbi was Producer/Director/Director of Photography for Steven G. Taibbi Productions, a television production company and a contributing editor at Videography Magazine for ten years, and he also wrote articles for other magazines. He's written television scripts, TV and radio commercials and was the lyricist for a song-writing team. He went on to be the vice president of Transplant Speakers, International and is now a public speaker and professional photographer. You may find out more about the author here: WhyImStillNotDead.com

CPSIA information can be obtained
at www.ICGtesting.com
Printed in the USA
LVHW012315180319
611112LV00010B/465